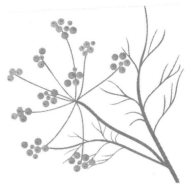

A Clinician's Guide
to Using Granule Extracts

by Eric Brand

Published by:
BLUE POPPY PRESS
A Division of Blue Poppy Enterprises, Inc.
1990 North 57th Court, Unit A
BOULDER, CO 80301

First Edition, June 2010
Second Printing, November 2012
Third Printing, July 2014
Fourth Printing, February 2016

ISBN1-891845-51-9
ISBN 978-1-891845-51-2
LCCN #2010907367

DISCLAIMER: The information in this book is given in good faith. However, the author and the publishers cannot be held responsible for any error or omission. The publishers will not accept liabilities for any injuries or damages caused to the reader that may result from the reader's acting upon or using the content contained in this book. The publishers make this information available to English-language readers for research and scholarly purposes only.

The publishers do not advocate nor endorse self-medication by laypersons. Chinesemedicine is a professional medicine. Laypersons interested in availing themselves of the treatments described in this book should seek out a qualified professional practitioner of Chinese medicine.

10 9 8 7 6 5 4

Printed at Edwards Brothers Malloy, Ann Arbor, MI
on acid free paper and soy inks

Cover and text design by Eric Brearton with Honora L. Wolfe

Table of Contents

*This book is dedicated to the inspirational teachers
who have touched my life—*

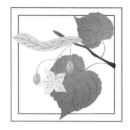

Preface

Over the past decade, granules have become the most popular adminis-tration form for Chinese medicine in the West. While granules are well-known for their convenience and portability, few Western practitioners have been adequately exposed to the diverse landscape of clinical styles seen in Asia. Consequently, confusion abounds on issues such as dosage, concentration ratios, and formulation strategies.

The world of granules is incredibly sophisticated, and practitioners in places such as Taiwan and Japan have been using granules for over 40 years. During my studies in Taiwan, I quickly noticed that Taiwanese doctors had a unique style of prescribing granules that was characterized by formula combining and consistent dosing norms. The Taiwanese method was different than what we tended to use in the West, which was based on a mathematical calculation to the raw herb dose weights.

Intrigued by the different dosing strategies and formulation styles seen between Taiwan and mainland China, I realized that even in the Chi-nese world there were few texts and resources for approaching the study of granules in a systematic way. With the exception of scientific literature related to plant chemistry and extraction techniques, few aca-demic titles exist to explore the clinical and cultural issues involved with granules. Most of the people with true expertise in granule manufacturing are associated with commercial enterprises or are involved in chemical constituent research; such individuals tend to have a knowledge base that is either highly specialized or potentially biased by their commercial ties. Likewise, most practitioners that use granules clinically have either been exposed to only the Taiwanese method or the mainland Chinese method, and few experts have pioneered academic exchange to compare the two systems.

As there are few strong primary resources for studying the culture of granule use, by necessity this text is not a scholarly work filled with citations and literature reviews. Rather, it is a practical summary of the experiences and conclusions of a single sincere student who traveled the world to learn more about granules. In the years that I spent researching the material that eventually became integrated into this book, I took many trips throughout Taiwan and mainland China to visit granule factories and interview clinical experts. From doctors to researchers to quality control specialists, I have tried to ask the right questions to the best experts that I can find, but I know that my work is still just scratching the surface. While I have learned a great deal along the way, I am always conscious of the fact that my current understanding remains incomplete and I am always humbled by the vast amount of knowledge that still eludes me. It is my sincere hope that this book will create a foundation for educated discussions about granules, and I look forward to the day when more knowledge experts publish works of great scholarship that correct my errors and make this small book obsolete.

I would like to thank the many experts that have helped me to learn about the art and science of granules. I owe a deep debt of gratitude to doctors that are living legends of clinical medicine, such as Feng Ye, Chang Hen-Hong, and Chang Hsien-Cheh. I am also very grateful to the industry experts that patiently answered my manufacturing and QC questions at factories such as Koda, KP, Sunten, Nong's, Guangdong Yifang, Tianjiang, and many others. My granule knowledge never would have developed without the expert guidance I received from these excellent clinicians, scientists, and scholars. Finally, I am grateful for the feedback and careful editing help that I received from the Blue Poppy team, as well as Bob Felt, Nigel Wiseman, Bob Flaws, Charlie Brand, Njemile Carol Jones, and Jocelyn Shinagawa.

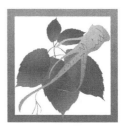

CHAPTER ONE

Why a Book on Granules?

Concentrated herbal extract powders, commonly referred to as "granules," are the most common delivery form for Chinese herbal medicine in the West today. Their widespread popularity is due to a variety of factors, chiefly related to convenience, consistency, and safety. However, despite their prominence, most practitioners have only been trained in the clinical use of traditional decoctions and often do not understand how to translate this knowledge into the effective use of granules. The aim of this book is to elucidate the clinical trends in granule use, with particular attention to challenging issues such as dosage and formula construction.

Most practitioners are drawn to granules because of the convenience they offer. Indeed, a full granule pharmacy saves thousands of hours of decoction time and fits into a space the size of a small closet. Granules also minimize safety concerns because they are tested for correct species identity, microbiological contaminants, heavy metals, and pesticide residues. The sophisticated lot tracking and other features of GMP (Good Manufacturing Practices) standards used in most granule manufacturing processes also improves safety and leaves less room for error on the part of the dispensing practitioner. In regions like Taiwan and Japan, the national insurance system covers granules rather than raw herbs precisely because of these safety features.

Patients often prefer granules because of their portability and convenience. Granules are easy to use and they do not require complex cooking instructions. They can be used without even having access to a kitchen and they minimize complaints about the odor of stovetop decoctions. In terms of value, granules are comparable to raw herbs and tend to be less expensive than other prepared forms of Chinese medicine when dosage is taken into account.

Researchers also tend to favor granules because they minimize confounding variables. A custom batch can be commissioned from a factory so that the exact same product is used throughout the study, and reference samples of the batch can be stored and precisely analyzed if the results in the study are promising. By contrast, raw herbs require authentication to verify their identity and they are less consistent in terms of their chemistry from batch to batch. When using granules for research, the natural variation in constituents can be harmonized by producing large, consistent batches and the identity of the source materials can be verified by on–staff experts.

Given the many of advantages that granules offer, it is not surprising that they have become the dominant delivery form of Chinese herbal medicine in the West. However, granules are used differently in different parts of Asia, and relatively few practitioners have been exposed to the trends in dosage and formulation styles that have emerged there. In order to gain a solid grasp of the clinical use of granules, it is important for Western practitioners to understand the different styles of use that make up the main evidence base for granules abroad.

At present, there are remarkably few reference books on the subject of granules, even in the Chinese world. There are major differences between the clinical trends in different regions, and these trends are poorly articulated even in the Chinese language literature. In Taiwan, practitioners are often poorly informed about the technology and trends in mainland China and the practitioners in the mainland have often had minimal exposure to the Taiwanese approach. Practitioners in the West often lack a strong understanding in the trends in either region, despite the fact that Western practitioners use granules with regularity. Thus, the initial inspiration for this book was rooted in bridging this cultural gap to facilitate understanding about the clinical use of granules.

This book begins with an overview of the granule manufacturing process. While the focus of this book is primarily related to clinical use rather than the technical ins and outs of production, there are a few

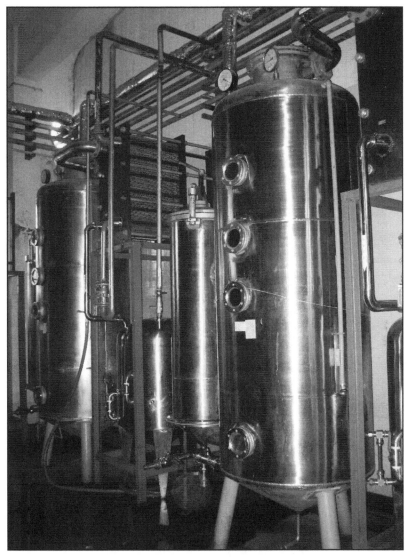

Figure 1. Evaporating machine to concentrate the water extract.

major issues in granule manufacturing that are essential to understand because they impact clinical reality.

In particular, there are significant differences in the way that granules are made in mainland China vs. in Taiwan and Japan. These differences are rooted in the prescribing style of each region, as well as the predominant method of packaging and delivery. Millions of patients have used granules in both the mainland style and the Taiwanese style, and both styles have ample evidence of their efficacy. Ideally, Western practitioners should understand these similarities and differences so that they can decide which style resonates best with their own clinical approach.

Different manufacturing methods utilize different concentration ratios and different excipients (inert substances added to improve the consistency of the finished product). Understanding concentration ratios is vital for proper dosage, and is an essential aspect of learning how to use granules. There are multiple approaches to dosage in the granule world, and understanding the factors that go into determining granule dosage allows us to be more confident in producing a reliable therapeutic effect.

Beyond understanding concentration ratios, dosage, and the physical products themselves, it is important to understand the different approaches to formulation seen in the Chinese world. In Taiwan, it is very common for practitioners to use multiple compound formulas together, while in mainland China it is very common for practitioners to build formulas from single ingredients. While the method used in mainland China is very similar to the method used for raw herbs, the method used in Taiwan represents a completely different paradigm and a novel clinical approach.

It could be argued that the formula combining approach seen in Taiwan is one of Taiwan's most distinctive contributions to modern Chinese medicine. In the West, many practitioners have used the granule products made in Taiwan, but remarkably few practitioners have been exposed to the Taiwanese method of using them. In Chapter 6 on formula combining in this text, the Taiwanese method of combining whole formulas together is explored in some detail.

In addition to examples that are characteristic of the clinical approach seen in Taiwan, I have discussed other approaches to formula combining as well. In particular, a modular approach based on combining concise base formulas is presented, along with tips on how these basic formulas can be combined and elaborated with single herb additions.

It is not uncommon to encounter practitioners in the West that are confused about how to use granules. Granules are a relatively new development in mainland China, and many teachers in Western schools of Chinese medicine were trained in China before the granule revolution gained momentum. At present, relatively few experts from Taiwan have come to the West to train practitioners in their distinctive local style, and relatively few Western practitioners have traveled to Taiwan to gain exposure to this style. Consequently, it is understandable that there is widespread confusion about how granules should be used.

This book aims to be an academic survey of the world of granules as well as a practical clinical handbook. Throughout the book, I have tried to pay particular attention to solving the challenges that many practitioners experience when using granules. I hope that my readers gain a better understanding of granule dosage and formulation strategies so that they can achieve superior clinical results. In addition to the body of the text, an appendix is included that can be used as a quick reference to common Chinese medical diseases and pattern–based treatments with granules.

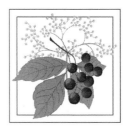

CHAPTER TWO

What Are Granules?

Granules are essentially a dry concentrated extract powder made from traditional medicinal substances. Generally speaking, granule products are made by replicating a traditional water decoction. Medicinals are boiled in water and the decoction is then concentrated into a viscous paste or a dry powder by evaporating the water.

This concentrated crude extract can be used to make a variety of different products, such as tablets, honey pills, or granules, and the pure dried concentrate can also be packaged directly in foil packs or gelatin capsules. The name "granules" can refer to the pure dried concentrate itself, but in actual practice most people use the name granules to refer to powdered concentrates that are made with additional excipients such as starch or dextrin to prevent the powder from clumping together.

Granule technology was originally pioneered in Japan for use in Japanese Kampo medicine. As the technology spread to other regions in East Asia, different methods of technology and clinical use emerged. At present, Japan, Korea, mainland China, Hong Kong, Singapore and Taiwan generally use somewhat different prescription styles and have different products on the market. To gain a comprehensive understanding of granules and their history, it is essential to understand the similarities and differences in approach between different regions.

In the West, granules from Taiwan and mainland China account for the vast majority of products in use. Most Western practitioners use a prescription style that is rooted in Chinese medicine rather than Japanese Kampo or other approaches. Consequently, this text is primarily focused on the features and clinical applications of granules as they are used in Chinese medicine. While a detailed assessment of Korean and Japanese granule use is beyond the scope of this book, I hope that future contributors will develop these important disciplines in the Western professional literature.

The Basic Process of Making Granules—Overview

There are significant differences in technology and approach from region to region and factory to factory when it comes to manufacturing granules. While the basic extraction method is similar at all facilities, the final product can vary significantly depending on what packaging form and excipients are used, as well as the sophistication of the extraction and concentration process itself. There is no single method that is inherently superior; each method of making granules has its own strengths and weaknesses. The ideal product for a given practitioner often depends on how they write formulas and how their patients actually consume the product.

At the most basic level, granules are manufactured by replicating a water decoction at an industrial scale. Stainless steel extraction machines boil the medicinals in water, and the resulting extract is transferred to a container that concentrates the decoction by evaporating the water at a low temperature. Once the extract is concentrated, it is made into a finished product.

The final stages of turning the concentrate into a finished product can vary significantly from factory to factory and product to product. By drying the extract completely, a pure extract is created. This extract, known as *jin gao fen* (浸膏粉) in Chinese, can be packaged immediately in foil packs or gelatin capsules. Without any additional excipients, the pure dry extract will tend to clump together if it is exposed to air and humidity. Thus, most products intended to be packaged loose in 100–200 gram bottles have excipients added.

Understanding Excipients

Excipients in granules are often called "fillers." Although the excipient (filler) is indeed an inert substance that dilutes the concentrated extract, the use of excipients is an essential aspect of granule manufacture. Most granules made without excipients clump together rapidly upon exposure to air and humidity, which dramatically affects the shelf life and convenience of the product.

While reducing the quantity of excipients is generally desirable in order to achieve maximum potency, excipients play an essential role in most granule products. The precise type of excipient used varies depending on the climate and the market preferences within a given region. Additionally, the method of ingestion affects the choice of excipient, since different excipients affect the consistency of the granules themselves.

Excipients in granules perform several important roles. Most importantly, excipients help the extract powder achieve a uniform consistency and prevent the powder from clumping together. The principle excipients used for granules include dextrin, starch, lactose, soluble dietary fiber, and cane sugar (usually only one of the above is used in any given product).

COMMON EXCIPIENTS USED IN GRANULE PRODUCTION	
1. Dextrin	4. Soluble fiber
2. Starch	5. Cane sugar
3. Lactose	6. Crude herb powder

Starch is the most common excipient in Taiwan. Taiwan's high humidity makes starch an ideal excipient because it doesn't absorb water as easily as dextrin. In addition, patients in Taiwan typically ingest the powder by pouring it into their mouths rather than mixing it in water. Thus, the Taiwanese market prefers a fine powder that can be poured into the mouth directly without being too sticky, and there is less demand for a completely water–soluble finished product. Large hospitals and clinics tend to use multiple brands of granules simultaneously in Taiwan, so most companies tend to produce finished products that have the consistency of a fine powder (called *xi fen,* 细粉) to ensure uniformity when mixing.

By contrast, dextrin is the most common excipient for granules made in mainland China. Dextrin is preferred in the mainland because it is more water–soluble. The use of dextrin tends to make a slightly larger granule, which is more appropriate for use in regions where the granules are taken by dissolving them in hot water. Dextrin is advantageous both because it dissolves better than starch and because it can be used in lower quantities, which means less inert material is present in the final product. However, dextrin absorbs water more quickly than starch so it is less desirable for use in hot, tropical climates. Dextrin–based products can often achieve higher concentrations than starch–based products, in part because the granules themselves form larger, denser particles. While this is desirable for patients who mix the powder in water, it is not preferred by patients who pour the powder straight into their mouths and chase it with liquid.

The vast majority of products used by Western practitioners of Chinese medicine use either starch or dextrin as an excipient. Other excipients are far less common on the Western market. For example, lactose is a common excipient in Japan but is not preferred for the U.S. market because of fears of lactose intolerance. Similarly, cane sugar is popular for OTC products on the Chinese domestic market, but it is not commonly seen in professional products on the U.S. market. Soluble dietary fiber remains relatively uncommon in granules, although it is widely used outside of the TCM industry.

Finally, crude herb powder made from either the ground raw herbs or the dregs from the decoction has been widely used as an excipient in granules in the past, though its use is now on the decline. Adherents maintain that using the crude herbs as an excipient is preferable to using a wholly inert material, but this method can be problematic in terms of heavy metal and microbial contamination. In the past, the use of crude herbs (or the dried, "spent" herbs recovered following the decoction process) was prominent in Taiwan, but is no longer very popular.

Understanding the Granule Production Process

While there are variations in the technology and approach used in the manufacturing of granules, the initial stage of extraction is largely similar from one facility to the next. The process fundamentally consists of the following stages:

1) Raw material sourcing and testing

2) Processing and slicing

3) Extraction

4) Concentration

5) Granulation

1. Raw Material Sourcing and Testing

Bulk medicinals are sourced from farms, wholesalers, and raw material brokers, often in quantities of 500 kilograms or more. Typical production runs produce between 50 and100 kilograms of extract powder, so it is not uncommon for granule companies to stockpile multiple metric tons of raw material for commonly used items. Given the large quantities needed and the significant costs incurred by testing the raw materials, sourcing is a key issue for granule manufacturers.

Ensuring the consistency of product from batch–to–batch is essential, and each manufacturer has in–house specifications that detail the quality, marker compounds, and other specifications for each medicinal that is ordered. Given the large quantity of substances required, establishing consistency in raw materials is essential.

In East Asian countries, granules are generally regulated as pharmaceutical products and must meet GMP (Good Manufacturing Practices) standards for production. Establishing the authenticity of raw materials is a basic aspect of GMP law, so manufacturers must verify that the materials used conform to scientific standards.

For most products, the basic reference standard is the *Chinese Pharmacopoeia*, which outlines standards for microscopy and organoleptic analysis as well as analytic chemistry (minimum constituents, specific marker chemicals, etc.). Organoleptic analysis refers to the characteristics of the substance that can be assessed with the naked senses—smell, taste, appearance, texture, etc. For most items in Chinese medicine, a trained expert can verify the identity of the medicinal based on its appearance, odor, and flavor, but a few items require microscopy or chemical analysis for definitive identification.

The *Chinese Pharmacopoeia* also outlines the standards for impurities (such as plant matter other than the medicinal item), ash content, loss on drying, and other specifications. In addition, the official pharmacopoeia of the destination for the finished product is generally used to verify that the levels of pesticide residues, heavy metals, and microbiology remain within the acceptable limits specified by the country to which the product is being exported.

For many items, companies have in–house specifications that help provide consistent quality control. This includes specifications such as minimum levels of marker chemicals or specifications on the production region or preferred species for a given medicinal. For the full–spectrum extracts used in Chinese medicine, most companies verify minimum levels of marker constituents for quality control, but they do not standardize the products to a fixed level of particular constituents. Thin layer chromatography (TLC) is used to verify the identity of a medicinal and high–pressure liquid chromatography (HPLC) is generally used to measure the quantity of its active constituents.

In other words, a company may specify that the ginseng that they use as a raw material must contain at least 5% naturally–occurring ginsenosides. Thus, when they measure their 3:1 extract, they expect to find a minimum of 15% ginsenosides in the finished product. In this example, the company is simply assessing the marker chemical to maintain quality control of both the raw material and the finished product. This approach is commonly chosen by companies that produce products for use in Chinese medicine.

By contrast, a "standardized extract" is a product that is stan- dardized to a specific constituent level. For example, a standardized extract that contains 15% ginsenosides would be expected to contain exactly 15% percent ginsenosides, no more, no less. These ginsenosides could come from any amount of raw material, and it is not uncommon for such preparations to have pure ginsenosides added in to hit the target quantity. When it comes to ginseng, it is not uncommon for pure ginsenosides to be isolated from the inexpensive ginseng tails, and these isolated ginsenosides can then be added in to enrich an extract made from lower–quality starting material.

Standardized extracts are popular pharmaceutical preparations on the mainstream market, whereas full–spectrum extracts tend to be more popular with traditional practitioners. Standardizing a preparation around a specific active ingredient creates a product that is similar to a conventional drug product. For example, white willow bark extracts can be standardized for naturally–occurring salicylic acid (aspirin), which allows the dose of salicylic acid to be easily determined. However, for products that have multiple active ingredients or unknown active ingredients, a full–spectrum extract that mimics the natural yield of a traditional decoction is often preferred.

Additionally, external testing requirements are often legally required by the government of the manufacturing country. For example, when using the herb Fang Ji (Stephaniae Tetrandrae Radix), manufacturers in Taiwan are required to grind and randomly test the mixed product from several different sections of the same lot. These tests must confirm the presence of tetrandrine and verify the absence of aristolochic acid, which ensures that the product has been correctly identified and is not adulterated with the toxic but similar–looking herb Guang Fang Ji (Aristolochiae Fangchi Radix). In Japan, the government requires constituent testing for Kampo formulas, which must conform to minimum levels of marker compounds for multiple ingredients. This confirms that the formula contains the correct herbs and ensures that the product meets a minimum standard of potency.

Typically, the sourcing expert for a given company identifies a desirable product and then orders a sample for testing. Once the sample has been tested for authenticity, potency, and contaminants, a large lot is ordered. When the lot arrives, it is randomly tested to ensure that it meets the same standards as the sample, and then the supplier is paid. Most granule companies have a standard operating procedure that allows them to easily reject raw materials that do not meet their standards.

Following manufacturing, additional tests are completed to make sure that the product has the correct consistency, stability, and potency. Tests for microbiological contamination, molds, heavy metals, and pesticide residues are conducted, and marker chemicals may be analyzed. Machines that simulate different environmental conditions are used to ensure the product's stability in a variety of different environments, and any additional required tests are completed (such as dissolution and hardness tests for tablets).

2. Processing and Slicing

Most granule manufactures do their own preparation for common items. Many items in Chinese medicine simply require honey–processing or dry–frying, which is usually done in–house. Granule manufacturers first wash the items and then they apply whatever processing is required, such as slicing, stir–frying, baking, etc. For example, Dang Gui (Angelicae Sinensis Radix) arrives whole, then it is washed, sliced, and may be stir–fried with wine for some preparations or left "raw" for other preparations.

When making formulas, granule companies tend to follow the specifications of the original formula when they cook the ingredients together.

Some items, such as minerals, are decocted for a prolonged period before other ingredients are added, and items that require specific processing methods (*pao zhi*, 炮制) have their *pao zhi* applied in accordance with the original recipe.

When preparing single extracts, usually the *pao zhi* form chosen reflects the method that is most commonly used clinically, or the method that is thought to have the best effect. For example, Shan Zhu Yu (Corni Fructus) is often processed with wine (*jiu zhi*, 酒炙) because this enhances the solubility of its active constituents and wine–processing has long been its traditional *pao zhi* method of choice. Similarly, Yan Hu Suo (Corydalis Rhizoma) is often processed with vinegar, which allows its pain–relieving alkaloids to become more soluble.

Other items, such as Yi Yi Ren (Coicis Semen) or Da Huang (Rhei Radix et Rhizoma) are used for different purposes when the product is processed vs. unprocessed. For these items, some granule suppliers thus offer a choice of more than one processing method. For example, one can order unprocessed Yi Yi Ren to clear damp–heat or one can order stir–fried Yi Yi Ren to supplement the spleen.

Items that require complicated *pao zhi* methods are often processed beforehand in special facilities. This includes toxic medicinals such as Fu Zi (Aconiti Radix Lateralis Praeparata) and Ban Xia (Pinelliae Rhizoma), as well as items that need to be processed before they are dried.

3. Extraction

The decoction has been the primary administration method in Chinese medicine for millennia. Most of the clinical experience amassed over the history of Chinese medicine is thus based on the water–soluble constituents found in medicinal substances. Although various non–decocted powders and pills have been used throughout the history of Chinese medicine, alcohol and other solvents have been used only rarely and in somewhat limited contexts.

For most products, granule companies essentially replicate a traditional water decoction. They use a large stainless steel, pressurized extractor that typically holds several hundred kilograms of crude material. After being processed and sliced, medicinals are placed into the extractor and covered with water. They are then essentially boiled in water and then the water is drained and concentrated in a separate set of machines.

Different medicinals require different amounts of water, temperature, and duration in order to get an ideal extract. The extraction time and temperature can be varied based on the medicinal that is being extracted. To determine the ideal processing method and extraction method for any given substance, granule companies often do research in a small–scale, controlled setting. In fact, specialized small extraction machines exist to mimic the large extractors for research and product development.

When assessing the desired extraction method for any given substance, a granule company must first investigate how that substance was traditionally used. Some items were traditionally taken as a powder instead of in a decoction, while other items were traditionally mixed with wine and taken separately. Items like San Qi (Notoginseng Radix) fall into the former category, while items like Mo Yao (Myrrha) and gelatin products fall into the latter category.

Items that were not traditionally decocted tend to have factors that limit their suitability for prolonged decoction. While most items used in Chinese medicine are suitable for concentrated water decoctions, there are a few exceptions that practitioners should be aware of. These exceptions can be generally categorized under the following headings: 1) delicate items that are easily damaged by heat, 2) resins and other substances that are not very water–soluble, 3) minerals, and 4) gelatins. I will discuss the dosage and clinical use of these items in greater detail under the following chapter "Understanding Concentration Ratios."

Delicate Items

Delicate items are substances that cannot handle prolonged exposure to high temperatures. Examples include San Qi (Notoginseng Radix), Gou

Teng (Uncariae Ramulus cum Uncis), and Da Huang (Rhei Radix et Rhizoma). Some items have different actions when they are cooked for a prolonged period of time. For example, prolonged cooking weakens the ability of San Qi to stop bleeding and the ability of Da Huang to free the stool, but both can be used to quicken the blood when they have been cooked for a prolonged period. By contrast, Gou Teng is thought to be relatively ineffective if it has been exposed to prolonged high heat, so it is generally extracted at a low temperature. Many delicate medicinals were traditionally taken directly as a powder rather than as a decoction, so their clinical use in granule form should reflect this fact.

For example, items such as Xue Jie (Daemonoropis Resina) are traditionally taken directly as a powder instead of being decocted. These items are generally sold by granule companies as a 1:1 crude powder rather than a true concentrated extract. Consequently, there is no need to adjust the dosage of these products because they are not concentrated and have never been traditionally used in decoctions.

Resins

Some resins, such as Mo Yao (Myrrha) and Ru Xiang (Olibanum), are not very water–soluble and were traditionally dissolved in wine. Overall, alcohol is rarely used as a solvent when making granules because most products were historically only extracted with water. However, alcohol is often used when making granules from resins. Interestingly, the use of alcohol as a solvent is restricted in Japan and Taiwan by law unless alcohol was traditionally used within a given classical preparation.

Minerals

Many minerals cannot be easily made into a concentrated form. The approach to minerals varies depending on the granule factory, but in general there are two approaches that are common. The first is to simply grind the mineral into a fine powder. The powder can be packaged directly or it can be mixed with dextrin, compressed, and packaged as a large–kernel granule. The second approach to minerals involves boiling the mineral in water.

Boiling minerals in water is the closest way to replicate a traditional decoction, but most minerals are not particularly water–soluble. Therefore, the concept of a "5:1 concentration" for many minerals is simply a method of satisfying perceived market demand. Companies simply identify the appropriate degree to grind the mineral so that 5 kilograms of crude minerals yields 1 kilogram of finished product. By grinding the mineral, some portion of it becomes suspended in water so that when the water is evaporated, the appropriate amount of mineral remains.

Both approaches to minerals have limitations that affect clinical practice. Simply grinding the mineral is problematic for items that are traditionally decocted because there is no way to precisely determine the target dose if a patient eats the straight powdered mineral instead of decocting the crude substance. For example, a decoction with 30 grams of Mu Li (Ostreae Concha) allows the Mu Li to interact with the other substances, and the patient ingests a relatively small portion of Mu Li after the decoction is strained. If the same patient takes 30 grams of straight Mu Li powder, it is far more than they would get in the traditional decoction because most Mu Li stays behind in the discarded dregs. It is difficult to estimate the equivalent decocted dose when the patient ingests the straight powdered product.

Cooking minerals in water is often regarded as superior to simply grinding them to a powder because this method comes closer to replicating the decoction process. However, the final product is often fundamentally unchanged from the crude substance, so it is not obvious that there is any significant difference between the two methods. Generally speaking, mineral medicinals are best in formulas that have been cooked together to replicate a traditional decoction. If minerals are used as single medicinals, there is often little difference between the crude, ground mineral and the same mineral that has been boiled in water on its own.

Another challenge in terms of minerals relates to items like Dai Zhe Shi (Haematitum), which contains a trace amount of arsenic. If boiled in a decoction, the patient likely ingests less arsenic than they would if they consume the mineral as a straight powder. For this reason, slightly toxic minerals may be more problematic if they are consumed as a straight powder instead of using them in traditional decoctions.

Without question, the best way to use minerals in granule form is to incorporate them into whole formulas that have been cooked together in the extraction process. For example, the formula Ma Xing Gan Shi Tang (Ephedra, Apricot Kernel, Gypsum, and Licorice Decoction) is made by decocting around 15–30 grams of the mineral gypsum with apricot kernels, ephedra, and licorice. If the premade granule version of this formula is given, the medicinals will be decocted together at the factory and the end product will be similar to the end product achieved in a home decoction. However, if the four ingredients are mixed from scratch based on single extracts, their ratio is entirely different because it is difficult to estimate the desired amount of the gypsum.

Gelatins

Gelatins are not traditionally decocted and they are not commonly found in a true granule form. Gelatin products, such as Lu Jiao Jiao (Cervi Cornus Gelatinum) and E Jiao (Asini Corii Colla), are traditionally crushed and dissolved into the strained decoction or dissolved in wine. If gelatins are boiled with other medicinals, they stick to the surface of the other medicinals and interfere with their extraction. The gelatin also clogs the machinery and becomes an unmanageable mess as it cools. In actuality, gelatins themselves are a traditional concentrate made by boiling animal hide, horns, or shells, and they cannot be concentrated further. Some manufacturers do sell "granule" versions of these products, but they are generally not concentrated. In fact, sometimes they are diluted because starch, clamshell powder, or powdered pueraria may be added to facilitate grinding. However, in most formula extracts, the other herbs are all cooked to make an extract powder, the ground gelatin being added to that powder during the final step of production. It is added at the same time as the dextrin or starch, it is never put into boiling water.

Additional Considerations in the Extraction Process

A. Modern chemical research

In some cases, modern research on chemical constituents influences the desired extraction method (as well as the *pao zhi* method). For example, Rou Cong Rong (Cistanches Herba) is an herb that has been traditionally used in water decoctions as well as in medicinal liquors. Its traditional processing method involves steaming it with wine, and modern research has found that some of its key active constituents are more soluble in alcohol than in water. Consequently, Rou Cong Rong is often extracted with alcohol in addition to water, making it an exception to the general trend of simply replicating a water decoction.

B. Steam pressure

The extractors used at granule factories contain the steam that is produced from boiling the herbs, which builds pressure and appears to increase the efficiency of the extraction. Increased pressure also allows the water to boil at a higher temperature if desired. Research has shown that some key constituents are more soluble under pressurized extraction, particularly flavonoids and alkaloids.

The use of pressurized extraction is relatively new given the long history of Chinese medicine. However, it is important to note that pressurized extractors have been widely used in Asia for decades with satisfactory results. Millions of patients in urban areas of China and Korea use herbs that have been extracted in small, pressurized extractors, and the majority of patients in Taiwan and Japan use granules.

C. Cooking time and temperature

Cooking time also plays a role in granule production. According to traditional theory, light, floating medicinals should be decocted for short periods of time, while sinking substances that target the interior are often decocted for longer periods of time. There are many references to this concept in the Chinese literature. For example, the *Wen Bing Tiao Bian* ("Systematized Identification of Warm Diseases") notes that the formula Sang Ju Yin (Mulberry Leaf and Chrysanthemum Beverage) should not be decocted for too long because its "flavor will thicken and enter the interior." The formula is meant to be light and floating to treat illness at the surface of the body, so the decoction time is short.

Medicinals with a short decoction time (such as items added *hou xia* or "at the end of the decoction") present a conundrum to granule manufacturers. To a certain extent, it is thought that many aromatic items were added at the end because the traditional decoction method rapidly disperses their essential oils via the escaping steam. In modern granule manufacturing, the essential oils are captured and reintroduced into the semifinal product. Thus, many items that were traditionally decocted for only a short time are now cooked for a longer period of time, such as Bo He (Menthae Herba).

Research is required to determine the best temperature or cooking time for any given medicinal. Research also allows companies to determine the ideal or maximum concentration ratio that can be achieved for any given substance, and it allows the company to determine how much water is required. It allows estimation of the ideal yield and allows manufacturers to predict the quantity of excipients that will be necessary to keep the product from clumping.

D. Formulas vs. singles

Replicating the decoction process for a compound formula essentially requires a relatively simple reproduction of the ratios and cooking instructions stated in the original source text (often a simple, uncomplicated water decoction). However, producing single medicinal extracts requires extensive research because each item has different chemistry and needs. For example, Qin Pi (Fraxini Cortex) was traditionally taken by a simple extended decoction, but modern research has shown that its active constituents enter the solution relatively slowly. Therefore, Qin Pi should be cooked for over two hours in order to make a high–quality extract; this discovery actually reinforces the traditional statement above about prolonged cooking causing the "flavor to thicken and enter the interior" (Qin Pi is used for internal disorders, usually affecting the intestines).

E. Capturing essential oils

Essential oil capture is a fundamental feature of granule technology. Essential oils tend to escape with the steam as the decocting water boils. Stovetop decoctions, as well as decoctions made in simple extractors such as Korean extraction machines, tend to lose their essential oils relatively easily. By contrast, granule manufacturers use a method of capturing the oils from the steam by retaining the steam in a closed circuit.

By cooling the steam, the essential oils condense into a solid state so that they can be captured. The essential oil technology varies from company to company, but most companies do collect the oils and reintroduce them into the semifinished product. Typically, the essential oils are added back in just before the product is dried, after the bulk of the water from the initial decoction has been eliminated.

5. The Concentration Process

After the medicinals are decocted in the extraction machine, the brewed liquid is strained out and collected in a receptacle. The liquid is then concentrated by evaporating off most of the water. This process is achieved by chambers that create a vacuum, which in turn allows the water to boil off at a lower temperature than normal (usually about 60°C instead of 100°C).

By lowering the boiling temperature of the water, the concentrating machines are able to eliminate thousands of liters of water per hour without subjecting the decoction to prolonged high temperatures. This process eventually yields a semiliquid extract that looks like concentrated, viscous goo, and the low temperatures preserve the flavor and constituents of the medicinals.

After the liquid is concentrated down to a thick viscous paste, it is called *jin gao* (浸膏). From this stage, it can be dried completely or it can be mixed with excipients and then dried. The different strategies used to make the final granules will be discussed below. If granules are not the desired endpoint, the *jin gao* can be mixed with liquids such as glycerin or alcohol, or it can be mixed with processed honey to make soft honey pills. *Jin gao* can also be used as a base to create tablets or softgels, and it can be packaged directly in gelatin capsules if it is dried completely (once the *jin gao* is dried, it is called "*jin gao fen*" (浸膏粉) if excipients have not been added).

To gain an appreciation for the process of making granules, try the following simple experiment. Take several pounds of Huang Qi (Astragali Radix) and cook it on the stove. Cover it in cold water and soak it overnight, then bring the water and Huang Qi to a boil the next morning. Boil it for about 4–6 hours, and then strain out the decoction and discard the dregs. This is basically the same as the extraction process above, albeit without the benefit of pressure and essential oil capture.

Next, take the decoction and put it back on the stove. Boil it down until very little liquid remains. Once it starts getting thick, reduce the heat and cook it very carefully so that it doesn't get burned. It will become thick, intensely sweet, and rich in color. This is basically the concentration stage, although the stovetop method lacks the ability to evaporate the water off at a lower temperature. (This concentrated liquid can be stabilized by adding alcohol and glycerin to extend its shelf life, but it is hard to produce a liquid that is much stronger than about 1g of crude drug per milliliter of finished product once it is stabilized with alcohol. One tablespoon would thus provide the equivalent of 15g of Huang Qi.)

If the concentrated liquid was dried (say, by pouring it into a pan and putting a fan on it), it would yield a dry extract. This is basically the equivalent of the pure dried extract known as *jin gao fen* that a granule company obtains by drying directly without the addition of any excipients. Regardless of whether a dry powder or a liquid concentrate is made, compare the concentrate made on the stove with a commercial granule product. The clean, intact taste of a good granule product usually surpasses a homemade extract, which is directly related to the capture of essential oils, the use of pressure, and the use of low temperatures for evaporating off the excess liquid.

While it is occasionally fun to make a stovetop extract, it takes a long time and it fills one's house with humidity and the smell of herbs. After making 10 extracts at home and calculating the material cost and the labor, one will look at the granule shelf with a whole new level of appreciation!

6. The Granulation Process

The final stage of making granules has the greatest variation in the manufacturing process. In general, the most common method is to spray the viscous, semiliquid *jin gao* into a drying chamber with starch or dextrin. This technique, often called flow coating, involves spraying a measured amount of viscous fluid onto a measured amount of starch. The paste binds to the starch and the bound material falls down a large chamber of warm air, forming a dry powder at the bottom. This powder is sieved and represents the final granule product.

The basic process above has dominated the granule industry for decades, and it remains the most common method in Taiwan and Japan to this day. In mainland China, this method is also commonly used, but often with some slight variations. Similar technology is in use in Korea and the U.S. as well, but on a smaller scale.

A common granulation method used in mainland China is to produce a pure, dry extract, and then add excipients such as dextrin. This extract mix is moistened, compressed, cut into small, coarse pieces, and then re–dried and sieved to form a large kernel granule known as *ke li*. Alternatively, dextrin or other excipients (such as cane sugar or soluble dietary fiber) can be added when the extract is still a viscous, semiliquid paste, which is then dried and made into *ke li* (large granules).

Types of Finished Product

There are a number of ways to produce the final granule powder. Four major product types are common on the market:

1) Loose granules made with starch, which often come out as a fine, aromatic powder with an even texture of small kernels. These granules have a good texture for direct consumption by mouth but they dissolve relatively poorly in hot water. This product is common in Taiwan.

2) Loose granules made with dextrin, which come out as larger, more irregular kernels that are heavier by volume and are generally less aromatic until dissolved. These granules have a poor texture

for direct consumption by mouth but they dissolve very well in hot water. This product is common in mainland China.

3) Granules packaged in sachets can either have excipients or they can contain pure dried extract (*jin gao fen*). In Taiwan, two sachet products are now on the market. One type contains the traditional Taiwanese granule with starch, while the other type uses a different excipient blend to create a product that dissolves better in water. In mainland China, the sachets can contain coarse granules (produced with dextrin) or fine powder, which is generally pure dried extract without excipients.

4) Loose, pure dried extract (*jin gao fen*) is also available on the market, but it is typically sold to manufacturers rather than final consumers. The pure extract powder can be packaged into gelatin capsules or used as a base for making other products, such as liquid concentrates, honey pills, or tablets. If the pure dried extract of most items is packaged loose in bottles, it tends to clump rapidly and become a solid mass. This limits its utility, so pure dried extract primarily reaches consumers in the form of gelatin capsules, tablets, and single–dose foil packs (sachets).

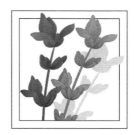

CHAPTER THREE

Global Trends in Concentrated Extracts

Japan

The roots of granule technology trace back to Japan. Japan was the first country to develop granule extracts, and Japanese technology and prescription styles have influenced other regions throughout Asia, particularly Taiwan. Joint investment between Japan and Taiwan gave rise to Taiwan's first granule factory, and Taiwan went on to dominate the Chinese world of granule extracts for nearly 30 years. The widespread adoption of automated decoction machines in Korea and mainland China caused the granule industry to develop more slowly in these two regions, but the past decade has seen a major boom in granule production and use, especially in mainland China.

In Japan, most use of granules is based upon either biomedical or traditional applications of classical formulas, which are often used in an unmodified form. The vast majority of the formulas used in Japanese Kampo were created prior to the Song dynasty in China (around 960 CE), and formulas from the Shang Han Lun and Jin Gui Yao Lue are particularly prominent in modern clinical use. Practitioners rarely build formulas from single ingredients, instead preferring to employ whole formulas or combinations of formulas. While few Westerners have studied Japanese Kampo itself at depth, the technology that was created to maximize the Kampo approach has impacted Western practitioners tremendously.

Granules are very strictly regulated in Japan. One must be an MD or a pharmacist in order to prescribe herbal medicine. Pharmacists cannot perform palpation or pulse–taking, unlike physicians. In addition, the products themselves must conform to very precise specifications. Kampo formulas are regulated like drugs, and any formula that deviates from the traditional historic preparation must undergo a process that is essentially regulated as a new drug application. For example, modifying a formula like Gui Zhi Tang (Cinnamon Twig Decoction) by increasing the amount of cinnamon twig would require a manufacturer to apply for a new drug permit. Safety and efficacy would need to be proven based on modern scientific standards, because the product would no longer be considered a time–tested, traditional drug product.

In addition to the laws limiting modifications in dosage and ingredients, Japan also has laws that limit the use of solvents that differ from those used in the source prescription. For example, a formula that was traditionally used as a water decoction must be extracted with only water. If a company wishes to use alcohol to extract the herbs, alcohol must be specified in the cooking instructions of the original classical source text (or else the company must apply for a new drug permit).

Japanese granule products are often packaged in single–dose foil packs. While the spectrum of formulas on the market is somewhat narrow in Japan when compared to the U.S. or Taiwan, there are a number of formulas that are particularly prominent. For example, Ge Gen Tang (Pueraria Decoction) is one of the most common remedies for the common cold in Japan, but this formula is almost never seen on the Western market. The presence of many classical formulas but comparatively few modern formulas is a distinctive feature of the Japanese granule market.

In Japan, classical formulas such as Xiao Chai Hu Tang (Minor Bupleurum Decoction) have become very famous for a wide variety of disorders, spurring an incredible amount of scientific research. Japan tends to have two main styles of Kampo in prominent use. One style is based on biomedical indications, and the other style is based on traditional diagnosis. Japan is a world leader in scientific studies and biomedical applications of classical formulas, and the modern branch of Kampo is currently making a major impact on global medicine. The traditional branch of Kampo essentially preserves a style that is based on early classical texts, and it is characterized by a strong understanding of disease mechanisms and an emphasis on abdominal and pulse diagnosis.

Regardless of the diagnostic method used, granules are much more prominent than raw herbs at this time. Patients in Japan typically take granules directly by mouth without stirring them into hot water. For this administration method, granules that are made into a fine powder with starch are desirable.

Quality control in Japan is generally very good. The *Japanese Pharmacopoeia* outlines very clear standards for each medicinal substance, and Kampo granule remedies also have clear specifications. The *Japanese Pharmacopoeia* sets very specific specifications for minimum quantities of marker chemicals in granule extracts, and manufacturers must demonstrate that their products meet these thresholds of potency. For example, a granule preparation of Xiao Chai Hu Tang (Minor Bupleurum Decoction) must demonstrate adequate marker compounds from licorice, bupleurum, and scutellaria in order to fit the specification guidelines.

Japanese Kampo fills an important niche in the global use of granules. This book is unable to do justice to the complex nature of Japanese Kampo therapy, so it is hoped that future authors will attempt to elucidate this remarkable tradition in greater detail.

Taiwan

Taiwan occupies a relatively unique role in the granule world. Granules arrived in Taiwan early on, and they have been used there continually for over 40 years. Taiwanese granule companies were the first to bring granules to the wider world, and many of the most well-known brands in the industry today hail from Taiwan.

Taiwan developed such a strong granule industry for several reasons. The close commercial exchange between Japan and Taiwan fostered the early development of a granule industry, and Taiwan's rapid economic rise enabled it to become a center for granule research and development. Liberal trade regulations allowed Taiwan to pioneer global markets early on, and the relatively high scientific standards in Taiwan fueled a movement to develop excellent quality control.

Japan has long been Taiwan's main customer base beyond the domestic Taiwanese market, and there is a bit of cross–fertilization with the granule methods between these two places. Both regions take granules directly by mouth rather than dissolving the granules in hot water, and both regions emphasize the use of compound formulas rather than single herb extracts. Importantly, the governments of both Japan and Taiwan also provide insurance reimbursement for granule products. This spurs a tremendous amount of growth and economic investment, and well as widespread clinical use and the experience that comes with it.

The Taiwanese method of using granules is relatively distinct because whole formulas are commonly combined together. With a repertoire of over 400 compound formulas on the shelf, Taiwanese doctors build complex combinations that boggle the young student's mind, yet there is nothing haphazard about the construction of a well–crafted Taiwanese style formula if one understands the approach.

Good doctors in Taiwan typically have a broad range of formula ingredients mastered, with a well–developed ability to see the relationships, similarities, and differences in each. A core formula at a higher dose often stands out at the center of the prescription, but instead of adding in just a few single medicinals to accentuate certain directions, whole formulas may be added in. The formulas are used as a single principle, much as many others would add a single herb.

There are several reasons why compounding whole formulas together has become popular in Taiwan. Given the Japanese origin of the granule technology and the prominence of combining classical formulas in Japan, it seems reasonable to think that some of the initial inspiration for creating a wide range of whole formulas and combining them to-gether may have been sparked by the Japanese influence. However, the most important guiding factor today is the widespread belief in Taiwan that formulas that are cooked together are clinically superior to formu-las that are created from scratch by combining single herb extracts.

Taiwanese doctors often compound two or three whole formulas to-gether, and they commonly add single herb extracts when customizing the prescription. Their insurance system pays for granule prescriptions up to a dose of six grams, which is usually given three times per day. Thus, most patients use about 12–18 grams of concentrated extract pow-der per day.

Although most of the granule products in use in the U.S. are made in Taiwan, relatively few Western practitioners are well–informed about the clinical approach to using granules in Taiwan. Since granules domi-nate the insurance–based healthcare system in Taiwan, doctors there have amassed a tremendous amount of experience with issues such as dosage and formula combining. This valuable information is just now starting to reach the West in earnest.

Without a doubt, the tremendous amount of granule use in Taiwan is re-lated to the fact that granules are the only herbal medicine reimbursed by the national insurance system. Granules are desirable for large–scale healthcare because they are well–regulated and hygienic, and each batch is tested and tracked. Granules are also well–suited to research because batches are consistent and traceable. Taiwanese patients pay very little out of pocket for granules and raw herbs are expensive by comparison. This has created an entire culture of granule use, with the vast majority of patients using herbs in a concentrated extract form.

Mainland China

Granule technology arrived much later in mainland China. Over the past decade, granules have become a major export product and have become very widespread in Chinese hospitals. However, the use of home decoctions and small extraction machines is still far more com-mon. Granules are only just now beginning to catch on.

The first thing that brought convenience to herbal medicine in mainland China was the arrival of small Korean extraction machines, which package decoctions in single dose liquid sachets. In Taiwan and Japan, granules were the first thing to revolutionize herbal medicine administration. By contrast, in Korea and mainland China, small extractors swept the nation and granules have only recently begun to catch up.

Granules first hit China in a major way after one major producer began supplying many of the large hospitals. Granules remain more common in large hospitals than small clinics, and they are often not seen in small pharmacies (with the exception of a few simple OTC products). At present, over 1,000 hospitals in China use granules. Despite the fact that granule use only accounts for a small portion of the total herbal medicine use in mainland China, the sheer number of Chinese patients makes the scale of granule use already enormous.

In contrast to Taiwan, doctors in mainland China tend to combine whole formulas together much less often, and primarily build formulas from scratch with single ingredients in a process identical to a normal raw decoction. While Taiwan has created a virtually new method of using herbal medicine based on their granule approach, granules in the mainland are largely an extension of the standard method of formula composition. In mainland China, whole formulas are less commonly available in a granule form, so nearly all prescriptions are made by combining singles. Rather than determining dose based upon a standard dose range of total extract powder, the dose is determined mathematically based on the raw herbal prescription.

While there are differences between mainland China and Taiwan in terms of their prescription composition when using granules, the biggest differences actually lie in their respective packaging and extraction techniques. In mainland China, granules are often packaged in single dose foil packs, which are sometimes called sachets. In Taiwan, granules are made into a smooth flowing powder that is dispensed from small plastic bottles.

The Chinese domestic granule market is growing very quickly. At present, relatively few whole formulas are available in loose granule form in mainland China, but there is a very wide selection of medicinals with different types of processing (*pao zhi*) available.

In Taiwan, many classical formulas are produced in granule form, but relatively few classical formulas are sold on the market in mainland China by comparison. Pharmacies in mainland China tend to carry a bewildering array of prepared medicines, each with its own custom–made recipe. However, pharmacies tend not to carry granules, and even the granule suppliers often do not make a wide array of classical formulas. By contrast, pharmacies in Taiwan offer little else besides classical formulas and singles in a granule form.

Korea

As in mainland China, granules are a relatively late arrival to Korea. Koreans were the early pioneers of the small extractors that came to revolutionize herbal medicine in China. The widespread availability of this versatile and convenient method caused granules to be less prominent in Korea than they are in places like Taiwan, where small extractors are only just now becoming popular.

Granule factories now exist in Korea. The technology used is similar to that used by their neighbors in China and Japan, and the quality is often excellent. The Korean granules tend to be soft, fluffy, and aromatic, and they dissolve well in water. Unfortunately, Korean granules are rarely seen on overseas markets, and their price is often much higher than the products coming out of mainland China and Taiwan.

In Korea, the most prominent method of herbal extraction relies upon small, pressure–based extraction machines. These "home extractors" are widespread in Korea, and they are a Korean invention that has had a dramatic effect on Chinese medicine worldwide. Their utility has caused them to spread outside of Korea, and they now dominate the landscape of hospitals and pharmacies throughout mainland China as well. Most of these extractors are essentially customized stainless steel pressure cookers, and they are generally paired with a packaging machine that dispenses the decoction into a durable, heat–stable plastic pouch. Korean–style extractors are currently in more widespread use than granules in both China and Korea.

Pressurized Korean extractors are essentially a home model of the pressurized steel extractors used in the manufacturing of granules. They can typically cook 5–30 packs of raw herbs per batch, and have been shown to significantly surpass home decoctions in the extraction of a variety of herbal constituents. The decoction is packaged without air so it has a relatively long shelf life even without refrigeration. In Korea, many patients regularly take supplementing decoctions in this form, and many pharmacies and even grocery stores sell pouches of ginseng and velvet antler extracts. Practitioners often prescribe a formula for several weeks at a time, and this delivery form is ideal for these customized, high–potency, long–term formulas. Because extractors can essentially make raw herbs convenient for patients, the corresponding formula composition style tends to parallel traditional herbal formulation approaches.

Generally, this is an excellent system. Prescriptions can be customized from raw herbs, and the traditional decoction process can be replicated with significantly less labor. Patients receive their decoction in single–dose, durable, heat–resistant plastic pouches that can be easily transported, re–heated, and consumed as needed. The pressurized cooking system allows for an extract that surpasses the traditional home decoction in terms of potency and efficiency, and the process reduces the human error of home decoctions in addition to providing convenience.

The efficacy of these home extraction machines has been well–demonstrated, as literally millions of doses have been taken by patients in mainland China and Korea using this method. However, despite their ease of use and efficient extraction capacity, the home extractors do suffer from a few limitations that are not shared by the commercial machines used to make granule extracts. For example, many home extractors do not have an efficient means of capturing volatile oils, which tend to be released when the decoction is released from the extractor into the packing machine.

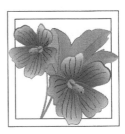

CHAPTER FOUR

Understanding Concentration Ratios

Understanding the relationship of raw herbs to the finished product is important when using granule extracts. The term "concentration ratio" is used to express the ratio between the source materials (the raw herbs) and the finished product; this is often abbreviated as S:P, which stands for the ratio between source and product. For example, a ratio of 5:1 implies that five kilograms of dried crude medicinals ("raw herbs") is concentrated to one kilogram of final product. This is also sometimes referred to in the herbal pharmaceutical industry as a 20% yield.

What Concentration Ratios Can Tell Us and What They Cannot

Concentration ratios are inherently useful because they allow us to calculate dosage in a meaningful, mathematically accurate fashion. A practitioner's greatest ally is a clearly–labeled, openly–expressed concentration ratio, because this information allows the practitioner to be informed about the amount of medicine that they are prescribing to their patient. Practitioners study dosage in the context of raw herbs, and most Chinese medical prescriptions are based on the amount of raw herbs that would be prescribed in a typical dose for use as a decoction. Concentration ratios are the bridge to understanding how much of a concentrated extract should be used to achieve an effect equivalent to a raw herb decoction, which remains the basic standard of care in professional Chinese medicine worldwide.

Concentration ratios tell us a lot about the potency of any given product, but ultimately the situation is more complex than the concentration ratio alone. While concentration ratios offer the most direct way of determining a target dose when using granules, it should be noted that there are many additional factors that must be considered beyond simple mathematical equivalence. For example, the cooking time, water quantity, solubility of constituents, and other factors influence the maximum concentration that can be achieved with any given medicinal.

Standardized Extracts and Liquid Extracts

Within the broader herbal medicine industry, we find several examples of different methods of calculating concentration ratios. This book is focused on granules, which are dry, powdered extracts, so granule products will be the focus of discussion here. Nearly all granule products used in Chinese medicine are full–spectrum water extracts. Thus, for the clinical application of granules, the only relevant approach to concentration ratios is a discussion of the source–to–product ratio mentioned above. Nonetheless, readers should be aware of the other methods of calculating extraction ratios that show up in the dietary supplement industry. Beyond the source–to–product concentration ratios that are used for granule extracts in Chinese medicine, we also see "concentration ratios" that are based on isolated constituents, and concentration ratios based on liquid extracts.

SOME IMPORTANT DEFINITIONS

1. Full–Spectrum Extract—An extract that captures the full range of soluble constituents. In Chinese medicine, full–spectrum extracts generally focus on water–soluble constituents because most products aim to replicate a traditional water decoction.

2. Standardized Extracts—Extracts that focus on specific marker compounds in a given product. This type of extract is common in Western herbal medicine but is relatively uncommon in clinical Chinese herbal medicine.

3. Concentration Ratio—A method of calculating the relationship between the raw herbal starting materials and the finished product, used for assessing potency and determining the raw herb equivalent for concentrated extracts.

4. Therapeutic Marker—Specific chemical constituents that are assessed for herbal quality control.

Outside of the world of professional Chinese medicine, one prominent method of calculating concentration ratios utilizes a calculation based on isolated constituents. These extracts are often called "standardized extracts," and their "concentration ratio" is calculated based on the amount of raw material that it would take to yield an equivalent amount of a certain therapeutic marker chemical. For example, standardized extracts are often made by mixing a full–spectrum extract with a fractional isolate (relatively pure active constituents that have been isolated from a plant source with the use of solvents and modern chemical techniques) in order to meet a specific ratio or "standard" for a specific product.

The use of fractional isolates is particularly common for items such as ginkgo biloba, which has relatively clear active constituents that require relatively high concentrations for an appropriate therapeutic effect. For example, ginkgo biloba extracts are often produced with organic solvents and standardized to 50:1 based on flavone glycosides and terpine lactones. Fractional isolates are more akin to pharmaceutical preparations than traditional herbal products, so they are generally not used within the TCM industry.

Some common Chinese medicinals such as ginseng are occasionally sold in standardized extracts based on a specific level of ginsenosides, but the standardized extracts found in the supplement industry are generally not used extensively by TCM practitioners. By contrast, the ginseng extracts that TCM practitioners use are often tested to ensure minimum levels of naturally–occurring ginsenosides, but the ginsenosides are not extracted with organic solvents and reintroduced to create a standardized extract. When ginseng is made into a standardized extract, usually large amounts of ginsenosides are extracted from the inexpensive leaves or rootlets with organic solvents. These isolated ginsenosides are then added in to a poor–quality extract of the root body so that the appropriate level of ginsenosides can be achieved. Most TCM practitioners do not use these products, instead preferring to purchase full–spectrum extracts of the root body (the traditional form of ginseng). The item preferred by the TCM community thus preserves the spectrum of constituents that would naturally come out in a traditional water decoction.

While Chinese medical practitioners generally do not use standardized

extracts clinically, most granule extracts used in TCM have been analyzed to assess their levels of marker compounds. Marker compounds,
such as ginsenosides, are used to measure authenticity and potency in
full–spectrum extracts. Here, the marker compounds are used as a reference rather than being the target of the extraction procedure, and the
main goal is to simply ensure that the starting materials are of adequate
potency for use.

Beyond the world of granules vs. standardized extracts, we also find
liquid extract products on the market that discuss concentration ratios.
Confusingly, the concentration ratios of liquid extracts are also often expressed by numbers such as 8:1 or 5:1, making the ratio seem similar to
that of granule extracts. While there are a number of ways that this ratio
can be calculated when taking about liquid concentrates, sometimes the
ratio simply reflects the degree to which the original decoction has been
reduced by evaporation.

When it comes to liquid concentrates, the most meaningful expression
of concentration reflects the amount of raw herbs per milliliter of finished product. Most methods of manufacturing liquid concentrates in
the TCM field max out at about one gram of crude herb per milliliter
(1g/ml, or about 30 grams per fluid ounce). Higher concentrations are
difficult to achieve because the liquid becomes supersaturated and
solids begin to fall out of suspension. This creates sediment at the bottom because the liquid cannot contain all the dissolved solids at room
temperature.

The Influence of Excipients on Concentration Ratios

The addition of excipients generally affects the concentration ratio of
granules and other delivery forms such as tablets and gelatin capsules.
Excipients are used for a variety of purposes, but they are primarily
used to improve the consistency of the finished product. Although they
have an important role, excipients affect the concentration ratio because
they dilute the active extract. As I discussed in more detail in Chapter 2,
the type and quantity of excipient varies depending on the manufacturing method and the delivery form of the finished product.

1. Improving Consistency

For loose granules, excipients are necessary because the extract powder will clump together without the addition of substances such as starch or dextrin. Without any excipient, the pure concentrated extract powder (known as *jin gao fen*) is difficult to work with because it is slightly sticky, very fine, clumps easily, and easily produces dust clouds when agitated. Typically, the granulation process combines the use of excipients with a sieving process to create granule kernels of a uniform size. The addition of excipients helps to create the right consistency so that the granule powder can be worked with easily.

It is possible to avoid the use of excipients if the granules are packaged in single–dose foil packs, but in actual practice most granules packaged in foil packs still contain dextrin or starch as an excipient. Although foil packs are extremely common in mainland China, many practitioners in the West as well as Hong Kong and Taiwan prefer loose granules to individual foil packs because the granules can be easily weighed and mixed together in any proportions needed, and the packaging is more "green."

Delivery forms such as tablets and "tea pills" require excipients that function as a binder. Typically, pill products contain binders and lubricants such as silica, starch, magnesium stearate, and lactose powder. Tablets and pills can achieve relatively high concentration ratios because they do not require large amounts of excipients, but it is essential to know the relationship of the tablets or tea pills to the raw herbs that created them. In some cases, finely–ground, nonconcentrated herbs are pressed into a tablet form; buyers must pay attention to concentration ratios when assessing tablet products to ensure that a true extract is being purchased.

For products that are encapsulated, the starting material can be either pure extract or extract with starch or dextrin. There is wide variation in what goes into gelatin capsules, because many granule companies simply fill capsules with the same product that is packaged loose in 100g bottles (loose granules require more excipient than the capsule delivery method requires, but it is often not practical for companies to produce separate production lines for their encapsulated products). Regardless of the starting material that is put into gelatin capsules, a small amount of excipient is often added to improve the smooth flow of the powder in the encapsulation machine.

2. Dilution

Relatively high doses are required for most items in Chinese medicine, and excipients are often minimized because they dilute the potency of the product. However, excipients are occasionally added to deliberately dilute the finished product, especially in the case of expensive or toxic substances.

Dilution with excipients is common in pharmaceutical drugs because of the high potency of many synthetic chemicals, but some strong agents in Chinese medicine are also diluted to improve ease of measurement and to reduce the risk of overdose. For example, one key Asian supplier of toxic medicinals in granule form dilutes the dangerous insect medicinal Ban Mao (Mylabris) so that one gram of extract contains the equivalence of only 0.1g of the original substance. This makes the dose easier to measure with a spoon and it reduces the risk of overdose. As with pharmaceutical drugs, transparency in labeling is the only way to truly manage such products effectively.

Some items, such as Gan Cao (Glycyrrhizae Radix) and Fu Zi (Aconiti Radix Lateralis Praeparata) can naturally achieve relatively high concentration ratios but they are often diluted because their typical daily dose is relatively moderate. Thus, while it may be possible to produce highly concentrated extracts of these substances, high concentrations become a nuisance when it comes to measurement. For example, if a 9:1 extract of Gan Cao is made but the majority of users only prescribe the equivalent of 3–6 grams of raw Gan Cao per day, the amount that must be weighed per dose is 0.33–0.66 grams of the 9:1 extract. In this example, diluting the extract to 6:1 makes it more manageable because the daily dose becomes 0.5–1.0g, a far easier number to work with in practice.

As mentioned previously, gelatin items cannot be concentrated. Gelatins are typically diluted when made into a "granule" form, because the gelatin must be mixed with starch, pueraria powder, clamshell powder, or a similar powdery agent that can be baked with the gelatin so that it can be ground. The traditional product E Jiao Zhu (Asini Corii Gelatini Pilula) is a pellet made by baking E Jiao with clamshell powder, and this same principle is in use when granule companies package powdered versions of gelatin products. Without a starch or powder to dilute the gelatin, it cannot be ground to a powder because the heat generated by the friction of grinding will turn the gelatin into a cement–like mass. Thus, gelatin products are often diluted in granule form.

Expensive items are often diluted to make the product appear to offer better value. Many herbs, such as Chuan Bei Mu (Fritillariae Cirrhosae Bulbus), Ren Shen (Ginseng Radix), and Tian Ma (Gastrodiae Rhizoma) are commonly diluted with excipients to reduce "sticker shock" when the customer sees the price of the product. (In the case of Chuan Bei Mu, many suppliers use either a low concentration of "true" Chuan Bei Mu, or a significantly concentrated extract of its close substitute, known as Ping Bei Mu. There is generally full disclosure of this on the Asian market but minimal disclosure on the Western market, because most Western practitioners don't know the difference and don't ask.) At present, relatively few companies openly advertise the concentration ratios of their products; there is significant competition to keep prices low and there is little reason to maximize the potency of the extract when a majority of customers do not ask for information on its concentration.

Variability of Finished Products

As mentioned in the section "Understanding Excipients," in Chapter 2, different excipients are prominent in different markets. For example, starch is the most prominent excipient in Taiwan while dextrin is the most prominent excipient in mainland China. Patients in Taiwan prefer to take the powder directly by mouth, and fine granules made with starch are superior for this administration method. Patients in mainland China mix the granules in hot water, so coarse, water–soluble granules made with dextrin are preferred.

In Taiwan, all granule products vary significantly in terms of their concentration ratios. While the items range from just over 1:1 to 17:1 or more, the majority of products in Taiwan come out with about a 3:1 to 5:1 concentration ratio. In Taiwan, most granules are made with about 50% starch as an excipient, though some suppliers use only 35% or so. Although there are a few exceptions, Taiwanese labels typically express the relationship between the raw herbs and the finished product very clearly on the label. Thus, consumers in Taiwan can determine exactly how much raw material is concentrated down to one gram of extract powder.

Interestingly, practitioners in Taiwan rarely prescribe granules based on their concentration ratios and the mathematical relationship of the powder to raw herbs. Rather, Taiwanese practitioners often use granules at a general daily target dose of 18 grams by weight per day or so, because Taiwan's national insurance only covers doses of 6.0 grams per dose (typically given three times per day to reach a total of 18g/day). At that dose level and with most products concentrated from 3:1 up to 5:1, this would give a patient between 54 and 90 grams per day when concentration ratios are factored in, depending on the company and the formula. Most Taiwanese TCM doctors have extensive experience with granules and they generally combine multiple formulas together. The prescribing style there revolves more around ratios of the different formulas in the total target dose rather than the raw herb equivalence. Because Taiwan uses a different dosing style and a different prescription style when using granules, the idea of using raw herb equivalence as the guideline to granule dosage never gained much traction there.

By contrast, most TCM doctors in mainland China primarily think about raw herb equivalence when prescribing granules. Whole formulas are not combined to the same degree as they are in Taiwan, and there is no single widely used target dosage based on insurance reimbursement. Consequently, the granule prescription style in China largely revolves around a raw herb prescription and its equivalent dosage in a concentrated extract form.

In mainland China, granules are administered in single–dose foil packs, with each packet containing the concentrated equivalent of a standard daily dose of a given medicinal. The concentration ratio of each product varies dramatically based on the solubility of the substance itself, and the weight of the granules in the pouch varies depending on the concentration ratio and the potency of the medicinal (a low–dose item like licorice would have less powder per pack than a high–dose item like rehmannia, even if the two had the same concentration ratio).

Overseas markets, such as the U.S., have a higher demand for loose granules than for single–dose foil packets. Thus, when mainland Chinese granule suppliers produce products for the U.S. market, it is common for the variable concentrations of the original starting granules to be evened out with the addition of more dextrin. Here, dextrin is used to dilute the products that have high concentrations to an even concentration ratio. The most common concentrations are 5:1, because most single herbs can meet or surpass the 5:1 concentration.

In this situation, the manufacturer bases the concentration ratio on a commercial decision. For consumers that dose granules based on their raw herb equivalence, dealing with multiple concentration ratios is a nuisance. Diluting the stronger items (6:1, 10:1, 8:1, etc.) to 5:1 allows for easy dosage calculations, and 5:1 generally works out well for most items.

However, some products, especially rich, oily, sticky substances and items rich in polysaccharides are difficult to concentrate to ratios as high as 5:1. Such items tend to clump together easily and they may lose their integrity and consistency if they are concentrated beyond 3:1 or so. Examples of such medicinals include Gou Qi Zi (Lycii Fructus) and Dang Gui (Angelicae Sinensis Radix). Unfortunately, many suppliers of 5:1 extracts do not disclose that there are exceptions that complicate the relatively neat marketing angle of consistent 5:1 ratios.

At present, lack of disclosure about concentration ratios remains an important issue. Suppliers rarely disclose the quantity of excipients and many suppliers of 5:1 extracts from mainland China do not mention the fact that a few agents are not able to achieve 5:1. Similarly, many Taiwanese suppliers do not disclose the fact that their products vary widely in their concentration ratios. Consumers are generally not well–

informed on the regional variations in prescribing styles and the issues that affect concentration ratios, so most consumers like to hear a simple answer like 5:1. Thus, many granule suppliers just state that the products are 5:1, even if they are not.

In an effort to solve these problems, more and more suppliers are beginning to clearly state the concentration ratios of their products. Some innovative companies have even taken to creating multiple tiers of concentration ratios for their products: items with high concentration ratios are done at a 9:1 concentration, items with medium concentrations are done at 6:1, and items that cannot be concentrated that high are done at 3:1. Such an approach provides a good balance, because it allows for open disclosure, minimal excipients, and ratios that are flexible enough to reflect the complex reality of single herb extracts and their potential concentration ratios.

Creating Consistency with Concentration Ratios

The natural concentration ratio of single medicinals can vary significantly from item to item. Items with more water–soluble constituents naturally tend to produce lower concentration ratios; these items are often sticky fruits such as Da Zao (Jujubae Fructus) or starchy substances such as Shan Yao (Dioscoreae Rhizoma). By contrast, many vine and stem products have a high crude weight relative to their water–soluble constituents, so they can often achieve very high concentration ratios. Examples include fibrous products such as Zhu Ru (Bumbusae Caulis in Taenia), Ji Xue Teng (Spatholobi Caulis), and Ren Dong Teng (Lonicerae Caulis).

Beyond the quantity of water–soluble constituents within a given medicinal, the characteristics of the constituents themselves affects the final concentration that can be achieved. Items that produce an extract that is naturally sticky or oily tend to require more excipient to prevent clumping, so these items tend to have a lower concentration ratio. Examples of such substances include Dang Gui (Angelicae Sinensis Radix) and Gou Qi Zi (Lycii Fructus).

Additionally, the quantity of water is important. As a basic rule of thumb, the herbs should have enough space in the decocting vessel so that water can circulate effectively. If the vessel is too densely packed with herbs or if the herbs are not sliced effectively to maximize their surface area, the extract is not efficient. To avoid this problem, good manufacturers conduct tests with varying quantities of water and raw herb materials in order to identify the optimal conditions for extraction.

Cooking time also affects the concentration ratio of a given preparation. At a minimum, the cooking time should meet or exceed the cooking time that is indicated for a traditional stovetop decoction. Cooking for prolonged periods of time tends to produce a more complete extract, and cooking the herbs a second time after the first batch of water is saturated will result in even more extract material (this tends to lower the concentration ratio because more extract is produced from the same starting material).

The question of what constitutes a "complete extract" or an "optimal extract" is challenging to answer. Some items appear to have active constituents that are best extracted with prolonged cooking. Other items are best with a shorter decoction time. Different companies research the ideal circumstances for each medicinal, but at the end of the day there is not absolute consensus on this issue, and little data is shared between companies. At present, there is a fair amount of consistency in the gross texture of products but widespread variation in their concentration ratios.

If the overall decoction time is shorter, the yield tends to be somewhat lower. If the decoction time is prolonged or if the herbs are cooked for a second time, more extract is created and the yield is higher. Thus, if ten kilograms of crude medicinals are cooked at a peak temperature for three hours and the resulting yield is one kilogram of dried extract, we say that this is a 10:1 concentration. If the same ten kilograms of raw material was cooked for ten hours with two batches of fresh water, the yield could be two kilograms of dried extract, creating a 5:1 concentration. Which is better?

Ultimately, in the example above, it is likely that there is not any one "right" answer across the board; it probably varies from substance to substance. Without question, it is essential that the extraction process replicate a traditional decoction. It would be ridiculous to cook the herbs for only five minutes before straining and drying the decoction, but in theory such a process would create very little extract relative to the raw herbs (the source:product ratio could be 100:1 or more). However, it would also be unnatural to decoct herbs for two days with several changes of water because such a process is not consistent with the standard decoction process of Chinese medicine.

When it comes to extracts, it is not about "getting as little out as possible" or "getting as much out as possible." There should be a balance between extremes that reflects the traditional decoction process. If the extraction is too inefficient, it is a waste of raw materials and it will result in a product that lacks clinical efficacy. On the other hand, if the extraction process is much more prolonged than a traditional decoction, the concentration ratio could be unnecessarily low, resulting in more profit for the manufacturer but less concentrated medicine for the consumer. Thus, the art is to mimic what should come out in a traditional decoction.

To use a familiar analogy, think about espresso coffee. Espresso connoisseurs prefer a relatively "short pull," meaning that they stop the shot before it is complete. The shorter exposure to steam rushing through the coffee results in a shot that is shorter and more concentrated, and it produces brown foam at the top of the shot called "crema." If more steam moves through the ground coffee, it will produce a larger shot that has more liquid and more solute but lacks the delicate "crema." If one dried out the espresso from a short pull vs. a long pull, the two pulls would have different concentration ratios because the longer pull will have more dissolved solids (solute).

If the short shot of espresso was dried and turned into an extract powder, we may find that a ten gram serving of ground coffee yields one gram of dried powder after being made into a "short shot" of espresso. This would be a 10:1 concentrate. The same coffee extracted with a "long shot" of espresso might yield a 7:1 concentrate, because more extract was created. Boiling the ground coffee in water for hours might yield even more extract, perhaps bringing the concentration down to 5:1. Which product would make the best instant coffee? With coffee, the short shot would probably have the richest flavor, but the cost per kilogram would be higher than the other batches because of the comparatively low yield.

Now, if Chinese herbs were as straightforward as coffee, it would be easy. Since coffee is only a single substance, it is likely that one could find the best way to extract it to maximize its flavor, value, and potency. However, each given Chinese herb has complex needs just like coffee does, and the process that is ideal for one herb may not be the best for another herb. Some herbs nearly certainly have delicate "crema" while others are probably best done by cooking them for hours and hours.

At present, there is a tremendous amount of scientific research that goes into determining optimal extraction ratios, but most of the research is done in the private sector. There is relatively little published data from neutral sources, so most of the current science remains in the realm of closely guarded trade secrets. Each manufacturer claims to have the best approach, yet each manufacturer also has the flexibility to accommodate large OEM (private contractor) orders that meet different specifications than their house standard.

Large–scale studies that measure levels of marker compounds would represent one of the most valid methods of evaluating manufacturer's claims, yet these studies have generally not been conducted on any comprehensive scale. Furthermore, if marker compounds were used as research standards for evaluating the quality of various products, the industry fears that the trend would create a strong incentive for manufacturers to manipulate their testing results by adding in fractional isolates of the marker compounds in order to make their products appear superior.

Consequently, there is no final word on which techniques are inherently best. Given the diversity of manufacturing methods, the varying needs of hundreds of disparate medicinals, and the inherent natural variations in plant chemistry, it is likely that there is no "one size fits all" solution to the question of concentration ratios. Rather than seeking out a single correct answer, it is important to understand the various issues involved, and the various perspectives found across the industry.

Taiwan

In Taiwan, both single extracts and formula extracts are produced at variable concentration ratios. The main prescription style in Taiwan can be regarded as a new direction in the field of Chinese medicine because it relies on combining whole formulas rather than building a formula based on single herbs. This style, along with the fact that the national insurance system in Taiwan limits the total prescribed daily dosage, has given Taiwan a new method of formulation that does not depend on converting granule weight to its raw herb equivalent. While this prescription style is an inherently valid, experience–based, and time–tested approach to using granules, few Western practitioners have been adequately exposed to this method of use.

As most TCM doctors in Taiwan do not use concentration ratios as their primary means of determining dosage, the Taiwanese domestic market tends not to use excipients to create even concentration ratios across the board. While the majority of products in Taiwan consistently contain 50% starch, the concentration ratio of the extract portion can vary widely from one brand to the next. In fact, sometimes there is close to a two–fold difference in the concentration ratio of the same product produced by two different suppliers.

This feature makes calculation to raw herb dose weights highly individualized from product–to–product, since one product may be 3.2:1 while the next may be 4.7:1. While computerized systems for precise dosage calculation could be easily implemented with these products, there is a lot of variability from brand–to–brand and sometimes even batch–to–batch. Since practitioners in Taiwan rarely use granules based on a raw herb conversion factor and the ratios are rarely provided on the U.S. labels for these products, few systems have been created to allow for easy dosage calculation based on raw herb equivalence with Taiwanese granule products.

Mainland China

As mentioned above, in mainland China it is common for manufacturers to produce most products at variable concentrations initially, and then the products are mixed with excipients to create an even concentration ratio (5:1 is the most common). This specification largely comes from market pressure to produce a consistent product that can be easily converted to its raw herb equivalent.

One common method used in mainland China to achieve this consistency is to add excipients in order to dilute the more potent extracts to an even 5:1 concentration. For items that naturally achieve concentrations that are lower than 5:1, the cooking time and other factors can be adjusted so that the yield is lower, or the product can just be naturally produced at 3:1 or a different concentration ratio. Some suppliers disclose these exceptions, others do not. At the time of this writing, full disclosure remains an issue with many manufacturers, in mainland China and Taiwan alike.

Whole Formulas vs. Singles

When producing whole formulas rather than single extracts, it is often much easier to create products with an even concentration ratio. While single herb extracts can vary dramatically in their concentration ratios, often these variations even out when a compound formula is decocted together.

Unlike single herbs, whole formulas are commonly made into prepared pill products such as gelatin capsules and tablets. Clumping is not an issue with tablets and capsules, so formulas sold in pill form can often achieve higher concentrations than formulas sold as a loose granule powder.

It is not uncommon to see tablet preparations that reach relatively high concentration ratios, such as 7:1. Pure extract powder packed into gelatin capsules can reach even higher concentrations. However, many products on the market that are sold in a capsule or tablet form do not contain any information on their concentration ratios, and some suppliers simply grind up raw herbs for use in pill products without using extracts at all.

In response to the widespread problem of prepared medicines that lack labeling information on their concentration ratios, many manufacturers have begun to produce products that have a consistent, openly–stated concentration ratio. It can be challenging for practitioners to dose prepared medicines if each remedy varies significantly in its potency, so it is common for manufacturers to keep an entire line to a consistent standard concentration ratio (5:1, 7:1, etc.).

In order to produce formulas at a consistent concentration ratio, it is often necessary to research the appropriate cooking time. For some formulas, boiling the decoction in water for just two hours may produce an 8:1 concentrate, while other formulas may need to be boiled for much longer to yield an 8:1 concentrate.

Generally speaking, the precise details of many manufacturing techniques are regarded as trade secrets. Despite the widespread use of granules, there is relatively little literature available to guide practitioners in issues such as concentration ratios, dosage, and clinical use. Clinicians tend to learn to prescribe granules from watching their teachers, and most of the people that have true expertise in manufacturing are biased by ties to private industry. A book such as this one is based on visiting many factories and speaking with experts in manufacturing and quality control, as well as interviewing numerous clinicians and observing prescription trends in Taiwan, mainland China, Hong Kong, and the U.S.. The field of granules is constantly evolving and replete with questions that are difficult to definitively answer, and our understanding is constantly being refined by feedback from other experts.

Examples of Granule Labels in Asia

成分	每公克中含有
白殭蠶 Bombyx Batryticatus	3.4g
以上生藥製成浸膏 Extract from Above （生藥與浸膏比例3.4:0.5=6.8:1）	0.5g
澱粉 Starch	0.5g

用法用量：通常成人一次服 0.4~1.2公克，
一日三次，食後溫開水送服。調劑專用。

Figure 1. Label from Bai Jiang Can (Bombyx Batryticatus). One gram of finished product contains 3.4 grams of crude Bai Jiang Can that is concentrated down to 0.5 grams of dry extract and mixed with 0.5 grams of starch. The dosage instructions suggest that adults use 0.4-1.2 grams per dose, three doses per day.

成分	每公克中含有
川烏 Aconiti Radix	5.5g
以上生藥製成浸膏 Extract from Above （生藥與浸膏比例5.5:0.5=11:1）	0.5g
澱粉 Starch	0.5g

用法用量：通常成人一日用量
0.4~1.2公克，調劑專用。

Figure 2. Label from Chuan Wu (Aconiti Radix). One gram of finished product contains 5.5 grams of Chuan Wu that is concentrated down to 0.5 grams of dry extract and mixed with 0.5 grams of starch. The dosage instructions suggest that adults use a total daily dose of 0.4-1.2 grams.

成分	每1.2公克中含有
麻黃 Ephedrae Herba	3.4g
以上生藥製成浸膏 Extract from Above （生藥與浸膏比例3.4:0.6=5.67:1）	0.6g
澱粉 Starch	0.6g

用法用量：通常成人一次服 0.4~1.2公克，
一日三次，食前溫開水送服。調劑專用。

Figure 3. Label from Ma Huang (Ephedrae Herba). Every 1.2 grams of extract contain 3.4 grams of Ma Huang that is concentrated down to 0.6 grams of dry extract and mixed with 0.6 grams of starch (final concentration ratio is about 2.8:1). Adult dosage recommends 0.4-1.2 grams per dose, three doses per day.

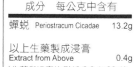

成分	每公克中含有
蟬蛻 Periostracum Cicadae	13.2g
以上生藥製成浸膏 Extract from Above （生藥與浸膏比例13.2:0.4=33:1）	0.4g
澱粉 Starch	0.6g

用法用量：通常成人一日用量
0.4~1.2公克，調劑專用。

Figure 4. Label from Chan Tui (Cicadae Periostracum). Every gram contains 13.2 grams of Chan Tui that is concentrated down to 0.4 grams of dry extract and mixed with 0.6 grams of starch. Adult dosage recommends 0.4-1.2 grams total per day.

【成份】**Ingredients** 每15公克中含有：
Each 15gm contains the following dry herbs:

人　參 Radix Ginseng	3.0g
龍眼肉 Arillus Longan	3.0g
黃　耆 Radix Astragali	3.0g
炙甘草 Radix Glycyrrhizae preparata	1.5g
白　朮 Rhizoma Atractylodis macrocephalae	3.0g
茯　苓 Poria	3.0g
木　香 Radix Aucklandiae	1.5g
當　歸 Radix Angelicae sinensis	3.0g
酸棗仁 Semen Ziziphi spinosae	3.0g
遠　志 Radix Polygalae	3.0g
生　薑 Rhizoma Zingiberis recens	2.0g
大　棗 Fructus Jujubae	2.0g
以上生藥製成浸膏　the above herbs yield an amount of dry extract	8.0g

(生藥與浸膏比例 31.0 : 8.0 = 3.9 : 1)

| 澱　粉 Corn Starch | 7.0g |

保存期限： **20070624**
Expiry Date
製造批號： **244241**
Batch No.

Figure 5. Label from Gui Pi Tang (Spleen-Returning Decoction). Every 15 grams contains 31 grams of raw herbs, concentrated down to 8 grams of dry extract. The dry extract is mixed with 7 grams of starch, making the final extract just over 2:1.

成分：每7.5公克中含有

白　芷(Radix Angelicae Dahuricae)	2.0g
甘　草(Radix Glycyrrhizae)	2.0g
羌　活(Rhizoma Notopterygii)	2.0g
荊　芥(Herba Schizonepetae)	4.0g
川　芎(Rhizoma Ligustici)	4.0g
細　辛(Radix Asari)	1.0g
防　風(Radix Saposhinkoviae)	1.5g
薄　荷(Herba Menthae)	8.0g
以上生藥製成浸膏	4.5g

(生藥與浸膏比例 24.5 : 4.5 = 5.4 : 1)

| 澱　粉(Starch) | 3.0g |

Figure 6. Label from Chuan Xiong Cha Tiao San (Tea-Blended Chuanxiong Powder). Every 7.5 grams contains 24.5 grams of raw herbs, which are concentrated down to 4.5 grams of dry extract and mixed with 3 grams of starch (final concentration is 2.7:1).

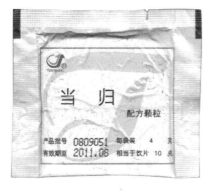

Figure 7. Label from Dang Gui extract. Every packet contains 4 grams of extract powder derived from 10 grams of raw herb. No excipient is present; the concentration ratio is 2.5:1.

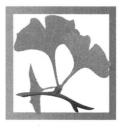

CHAPTER FIVE

Dosing Guidelines for Granule Products

Invariably, dosage is a challenging issue for practitioners who are new to the use of granules. Dosage of granules is a complex issue, and there are multiple styles of approach. In Taiwan and Japan, it is common to combine whole formulas and in mainland China and Western countries it is common to mix formulas from single herb extracts. Each regional style has variations in the way that products are combined and dosed.

There is no final consensus on the best way to dose granule products. There are several global trends to consider, and several different strategies that should be understood. Once we understand the issues involved and the dosing precedents that have been widely used clinically, it is not difficult to dose granule products. As with raw decoctions, dosage depends on many factors, such as the constitution of the patient, the severity of the illness, the potency of the individual herbs used, and the clinical training of the practitioner.

Understanding the Basics with Loose Granules

Many practitioners in Taiwan use granules in six–gram doses, which are given three times per day. This gives a total daily dosage of about 18 grams by weight.[1] It is also common to see prescriptions that contain only 3–4 grams per dose, so ultimately the standard daily dose in Taiwan could be said to range from about 10–18 grams per day. By using a total daily target dose, it is possible to easily determine the ratio of individual ingredients necessary to reach this target dose.

If one is mixing a formula from loose granules that are single medicinal extracts, a total target dose of around 10–18 grams per day is usually considered suitable for most cases. The dosage of each individual medicinal tends to vary based on its potency and nature. Most single medicinals tend to be used at a dose range of 0.5–3.0 grams per day (about 1–1.5g/day for most average items seems to work well).

If one is prescribing a classical formula without modification, around 8–15 grams per day is generally appropriate, depending on the number of ingredients within the formula and the clinical presentation of the patient. Formulas with more ingredients call for a higher total daily dose, whereas small formulas with few ingredients utilize lower daily doses. If a whole formula is used to modify a prescription (representing an auxiliary aspect of treatment rather than being the main thrust of the treatment), it is common for a granule formula to be added in at a dose of 3–6 grams per day.

Often, this dose range is mathematically a bit lower than the corresponding raw herbal dosage, but the increased efficiency of extraction that a controlled setting provides generally allows for a slight reduction in overall raw material weight. Additionally, other factors play a major role in determining dosage, such as the intensity of the case and the number of ingredients in the formula, as well as the potency of the herbs and the relative emphasis of their principles.

Just like when using raw medicinals by decoction, if you are mixing a formula from loose granules, each item has its own dose range when prescribed as a granule extract. It can be useful to group the items into

---

[1] In this text, wherever I use a gram measurement, I am discussing the grams used *by weight*, *not* the amount the patient is receiving by the extract's concentration ratio. This is because each company's products vary widely in concentration.

low, middle, and high dose ranges, though one's thinking should always be flexible in response to the case.

Items that are potent by weight and have a lower standard dose range are often prescribed in doses of 0.5g/day or even 0.3g/day; examples include items such as Rou Gui (Cinnamomi Cortex) or Wu Zhu Yu (Evodiae Fructus). Items that are used in raw dose weights of 3–6 grams are usually used in a relatively low granule dose range, such as 0.3–0.5 grams per day.

Average items are often used at a dose of 1.0–1.5g/day. Most average items that are used at this midrange are prescribed raw in decoction formulas at doses of about 6–15 grams. Examples include Bai Shao (Paeoniae Radix Alba), Bai Zhu (Atractylodis Macrocephalae Rhizoma), and Fu Ling (Poria).

Medicinals that are weak by weight require larger doses, often 2–3 grams of granules per day or even more. These items tend to be used by decoction in doses of 10–30 grams. Examples include Yi Yi Ren (Coicis Semen), Mu Li (Ostreae Concha), and Shan Yao (Dioscoreae Rhizoma).

Dealing With Items That May Not Be Concentrated

As mentioned in Chapter 2 in the section on extraction techniques, some items cannot be concentrated. Although many of these items are stocked by granule suppliers, many companies sell them as ground powder rather than a concentrate. The reason that a given item cannot be concentrated varies depending on the medicinal, and its dosage in granule preparations always depends on the traditional method and dosage of the substance itself.

When prescribing these medicinals, one must generally choose whether or not to preserve their traditional dosage in the granule form. Many of these items were traditionally regarded as being less effective in decoctions, so they were historically taken as a powder. Since most of them have a moderate dose range of 1–3 grams, they can easily be taken at this same traditional dose along with other granules.

For items that were traditionally used at higher doses, such as gelatins, we have to make a choice. We can either increase the size of the total granule prescription dramatically to accommodate the traditional dose, or we can use a lower than normal dose of the nonconcentrated item. The latter choice is often used when cost is a factor in the treatment; cost is sometimes an outside constraint that complicates any clinical decision–making process.

Below are several medicinals that are commonly sold in a nonconcentrated form. To understand their use, it is best to consider them on a case–by–case basis.

San Qi (Notoginseng Radix)

San Qi (Notoginseng Radix) has delicate constituents that are damaged by heat, so prolonged cooking negatively impacts its blood–stanching ability. It was traditionally considered best when taken as a powder to stanch bleeding, so a 1:1 (nonconcentrated) product can be used at a dose of about 1–3 grams. In fact, 1–3 grams is the same dose that would be traditionally taken as a ground powder.

Alternatively, San Qi can be decocted in water and concentrated at a low temperature. It can reach concentrations of 6:1 or more by this method. The concentrated product can be used at a lower dose range than the simple ground powder, so it is important to know whether a given San Qi product is crude powder or an extract. When decocted, the traditional dose of San Qi was 3–9 grams, which is higher than its dose range as a powder (1–3 grams). Crude powder may have a stronger ability to stop bleeding, but the blood–quickening action of the concentrated product is probably more potent by weight.

Chuan Bei Mu (Fritillariae Cirrhosae Bulbus)

Chuan Bei Mu (Fritillariae Cirrhosae Bulbus) is often too expensive to make a granule extract affordable. Various products from related species (thought to have similar actions) are often used as substitutes when preparing concentrates. Most companies supply either a 1:1 (non–concentrated) powder of true Chuan Bei Mu or a concentrated extract of its close relative Ping Bei Mu (Bulbus Fritillariae Ussuriensis).

Ping Bei Mu is a common substitute for Chuan Bei Mu. Most of the "Chuan Bei Mu" on both the raw and granule market is actually Ping Bei Mu, which has a slightly different shape. The two are listed as two separate medicinals in the Chinese Pharmacopoeia, but they are ascribed the same functions and are traditionally used in a similar fashion. It takes expertise to tell Chuan Bei Mu and Ping Bei Mu from one another, and the two products are both generally regarded as Chuan Bei Mu. True Chuan Bei Mu is considered the top quality and Ping Bei Mu is considered as midgrade "Chuan Bei Mu."

When using Chuan Bei Mu in granule form, attention should be paid to whether the product is a ground powder (1:1) or a concentrated extract (which can reach 6:1 or more). The pure powder should be taken at a dose of 1–3 grams, while the extract can be used at a dose of 1.0–1.5 grams.

Xi Yang Shen (Panacis Quinquefolii Radix)

Xi Yang Shen (Panacis Quinquefolii Radix) is also often sold as a crude ground powder because of its expense. Like Chuan Bei Mu (Fritillariae Cirrhosae Bulbus), Xi Yang Shen can be traditionally taken as a powder as well as in a decoction, so both straight powder and extracts are appropriate.

If Xi Yang Shen is being used as a straight powder, it should be taken at a dose of 1–3 grams. If it is used as a concentrated extract, doses of 0.5–1.5 grams are generally considered appropriate (it typically is sold at a concentration ratio of 3:1 to 6:1).

When using Xi Yang Shen in "granule" form, it is best to first assess whether the product in use is a true granule extract or simply a crude powder, because both are widespread on the market. For example, the Taiwan domestic market does not have Xi Yang Shen in granule form, but many Taiwan–based companies sell Xi Yang Shen in their granule line in the U.S.. Some of these products are extracts and some are simply the ground crude herb; it is important to be sure what product is being dispensed so that it can be dosed appropriately.

Gelatins

E Jiao (Asini Corii Colla), Gui Ban Jiao (Testudinis Carapacis et Plastri Gelatinum), Lu Jiao Jiao (Cervi Cornus Gelatinum), and Bie Jia Jiao (Trionycis Caparacis Gelatinum) are animal gelatin products. For reasons explained earlier, they cannot be concentrated because they are effectively already concentrated substances. Further boiling just causes them to stick like glue in the machines, and their traditional use was as a powder that is mixed into warm wine or a decoction.

Gelatin products are commonly given in relatively high doses, sometimes 10 grams or more. When using these products in a granule form, a large dose of 10 grams is usually added separately. If a patient takes 18 grams per day of total granules, a full strength dose of a gelatin product like E Jiao can easily take up half of the dose. In order to prevent a single medicinal from dominating the prescription and limiting the amount of other herbs that can fit into the 18 gram daily dose, some practitioners use the gelatin product in a lower dose than normal (often 1–3 grams per day).

In some situations, there are limits to the total amount of granules that can be prescribed based on outside factors. For example, doctors in Taiwan can only prescribe granules in doses of up to six grams because of limits on insurance reimbursement. This six gram dose is generally given three times per day, but it limits the amount of total granules that can be easily prescribed. If a doctor chooses to use a gelatin addition such as E Jiao, the doctor must choose how much to prescribe. If a full–strength dose of 10 grams is given, there will be only eight grams remaining for all the other medicinals. If a two gram dose of E Jiao is given, it doesn't compromise the dosage of the other medicinals in the formula, but it is below the ideal dose range for E Jiao itself.

If there is no financial limit to the total amount of granules that can be prescribed, then the most traditional approach would call for a high dose of the gelatin product and a standard, full–strength dose of everything else. However, it is common for granules to be sold by weight at a significant markup, so using high doses of gelatin products can drive up the price of a prescription. Consequently, many practitioners use gelatins in low doses in granule preparations (1–3g), even if they would ordinarily use gelatins in high doses (6–15g) when taken with decoctions.

Lu Rong (Cervi Cornu Pantotrichum)

Lu Rong (Cervi Cornu Pantotrichum) is a very expensive medicinal. True Lu Rong is derived from deer antler that is harvested early in the season, when its surface is covered in soft velvet and the antler is not fully mature. Lu Rong has many different grades and qualities, and it is traditionally taken as a powder more frequently than it is used by decoction.

As a powder of the crude medicinal, Lu Rong is used at a dose range of 1–3 grams. Thus, it is potent enough to be used in a crude, nonconcentrated form. If Lu Rong was made into a concentrated extract, it would be very expensive because the raw material cost is extremely high. Premium quality Lu Rong in a concentrated extract form would be too expensive for most customers to consider, so many companies instead produce extracts of Lu Jiao (Cervi Cornu) instead. Lu Jiao is the mature antler, which is much cheaper than Lu Rong.

Unfortunately, at the time of this writing, Lu Jiao and Lu Rong are poorly differentiated on the granule market in Western countries such as the U.S.. Most practitioners are familiar with the name Lu Rong but not the name Lu Jiao, so they seek the product under the name Lu Rong. Manufacturers typically produce an extract from Lu Jiao and then sell it as Lu Rong to meet the customer demand, but ultimately this practice is less than ideal in terms of honest representation. Lu Rong is a delicate, expensive medicinal that is very powerful, while Lu Jiao is a comparatively inexpensive substitute. While the two have similar indications, Lu Jiao is much weaker (though it has an additional action of quickening the blood to treat injuries).

When purchasing Lu Rong as a granule product, be sure to ask whether the product is true Lu Rong or whether it is Lu Jiao instead. Lu Jiao is often available as an extract of 5:1 or higher, and it can be used in a dose of 0.5–3.0 grams per day. True Lu Rong is almost never seen on the granule market, but in theory it could be used at a dose of 0.3–1.0 gram per day. As a powder of the crude medicinal, Lu Rong is used at a dose of 1–3 grams.

Chen Xiang (Aquilariae Lignum Resinatum)

Chen Xiang (Aquilariae Lignum Resinatum) is often not concentrated, due to its rarity and expense. Chen Xiang is a resinous wood that is very valuable and commonly substituted with inexpensive, young wood or counterfeit products. Extracts of Chen Xiang exist on the market, but many suppliers do not indicate whether the product is a ground crude substance or an extract on the label.

As a ground crude substance, quality Chen Xiang is highly aromatic. It is potent enough to be a viable medicinal without being made into a concentrate, and the traditional method of taking Chen Xiang is to use 1–3 grams of the crude substance as a powder.

Premium quality Chen Xiang is never made into a concentrated extract. It is already very valuable as a crude medicinal and it would be astronomically expensive if it was made into a concentrated extract. If high quality Chen Xiang is used, it is invariably sold as a 1:1 (nonconcentrated) powder. If Chen Xiang is made into a concentrated extract, younger, less resinous wood is almost always used.

For extracts of Chen Xiang, 1–3 grams per day is a typical dose. High quality Chen Xiang can also be used as a powder in doses of 1–3 grams. While the dosage is similar depending on whether the premium product or the concentrated extract of the young wood is used, the premium product is generally considered superior. Both products can be relatively expensive, but the truly premium crude product can easily be inaccessible due to its rarity and expense.

On the raw herb market, counterfeit Chen Xiang products abound, so even a granule product made from the young wood can be a good choice for practitioners that are not trained in issues of quality discernment.

Ge Jie (Gecko)

Ge Jie (Gecko) is also very rarely seen as a concentrate because of its expense. Some Chinese manufacturers offer it as a 2:1 concentrate, but it is rarely seen on the Western market and is almost never seen on the Taiwan domestic market. Most suppliers in the West carry a Ge Jie product, but it is typically just the ground crude medicinal rather than an extract.

If Ge Jie is used, it can be ground and administered as a crude medicinal. The skin, head, and claws should be removed and the use of the tail should be maximized. If the crude substance is used, a dose of 1–3 grams as a powder is sufficient. If a granule extract is used, a dose of 0.5–2.0 grams is adequate.

Xue Jie (Daemonoropis Resina)

Xue Jie (Daemonoropis Resina) is a resin that is rarely used in a concentrated form. It is not very water–soluble, and it is often sold as a crude powder rather than as a true granule extract. Traditionally, Xue Jie was taken directly as a powder rather than as a decoction, so its traditional dose range of 1–3 grams as a powder remains intact when using it with granule products.

At present, concentrated forms of Xue Jie do not seem to be available, so it should be assumed that most Xue Jie products simply contain the ground crude substance. In some cases, excipients are added to produce the granule product; at least one product on the market is actually 0.5:1 in terms of its concentration ratio.

Hu Po (Succinum)

Hu Po (Succinum) is another resin that is difficult to concentrate. It was traditionally taken as a powder in doses of 1–3 grams. Many suppliers sell Hu Po as a crude powder, though it is sometimes sold as a concentrate at 2:1 or higher. Generally speaking, extracts should use 0.5–2.0 grams, while the crude substance should be used at a dose of 1–3 grams.

Ru Xiang (Olibanum) and Mo Yao (Myrrha)

Ru Xiang (Olibanum) and Mo Yao (Myrrha) are not very water–soluble, so they are often sold as a ground powder. Alternatively, they can be concentrated by using alcohol as a solvent. Wine was traditionally used to dissolve these two products, so the use of alcohol is considered acceptable with these two substances.

When alcohol is used, the concentration ratio can be as high as 8:1 to 12:1 for these substances. Concentrated granules can thus be used at a dose of 0.5–1.0 grams per day, or slightly higher if the granules are concentrated to 5:1 (1.0–2.0 grams can be used). For products that are not extracts, the dose should be 3–9 grams.

Minerals

Many minerals present a challenge in terms of dosage. It is difficult to concentrate many medicinals because they are often not very water soluble. Concentration ratios for minerals vary dramatically; some manufacturers sell products that are the pure ground mineral (1:1) while others sell water extracts that are listed as 20:1 or even 30:1. Often, water extracts simply replicate the traditional decoction process and obtain a "yield" based on the particles of ground minerals that become suspended in the water. Many minerals are left unchanged by the decoction process, so it is difficult to tell what dose is ideal.

When decocting mineral substances with other medicinals, most of the mineral itself stays behind in the dregs of the decoction. Only a small portion of the total mineral dose is actually ingested by the patient. When minerals are given in granule form, the entire substance is ingested. Thus, it is difficult to fully replicate the decoction experience when using minerals in granule form, unless the minerals are incorporated into a whole granule formula that has been decocted together.

Compound granule formulas are the most desirable way to use mineral products in granule form, because the minerals are decocted with the other ingredients. In compound formulas, whatever interactions exist with the minerals and the other substances are maintained, and whatever dissolved minerals the patient would ingest with a traditional decoction will be present in a similar proportion in the granule product.

There is not a true consensus about how much of a single granule mineral should be used to approximate a decoction. For example, it is difficult to replicate a formula such as Ma Xing Gan Shi Tang (Ephedra, Apricot Kernel, Licorice, and Gypsum Decoction) by mixing single medicinals, because it is difficult to estimate how much Shi Gao (Gypsum Fibrosum) should added to mimic the traditional decoction. This issue is a key topic of academic and clinical debate, but there is no final answer that everyone agrees with. While granules have been around long enough to have proven their efficacy, they are still a somewhat new development in Chinese medicine, and there remains a lack of consensus on issues such as the proper dosage of minerals.

Overall, most practitioners seem to use between 1–3 grams of mineral agents per day in granule prescriptions. A range of 1–3 grams per day for minerals is quite common when using granule products in Taiwan, mainland China, and the U.S., so this quantity seems to strike a moderate balance that is anecdotally successful in clinic.

Main Approaches to Granule Dosage

In general, dosage trends can be divided into two main styles:

1) Dosage as a mathematical relationship between the raw herbs and the extract

    Mainland Chinese approach

    Sachets

    5:1 Extracts

    3:1, 6:1, 9:1 Extracts

2) Dosage based on clinical experience with common dose ranges

    Dosage styles in Taiwan

    Dosage styles in the West

In mainland China, granules are generally dosed to replicate the equivalent amount of raw medicinals that would be used by decoction. Most Chinese hospitals use single–dose sachets with variable concentration ratios, but many Chinese granules sold in overseas markets are concentrated to 5:1. Recently, new products have begun to arrive that have multiple tiers of concentration, such as 3:1, 6:1, and 9:1. As long as the concentration ratio is openly stated, these products can all be very accurately used to determine dosage based on raw herb equivalence.

In Taiwan, forty years of collective experience using set dosage limits and formula combining has evolved a new style of dosage and clinical use. The Taiwanese method stands out in contradistinction to the mainland Chinese method because it varies in its dosage and method of formulation. Both regions use the same fundamental Chinese medicine theory, but they use slightly different granule products and clinical styles. Most notably, as mentioned above, practitioners in Taiwan combine whole formulas together frequently, with single–medicinal additions.

In the West, a mixture of cultural influences has created an eclectic, varied approach. Many Western practitioners combine single extracts and formulate granule prescriptions in a way that parallels raw herb decoctions, so it could be said that the Western style is similar to the style used in mainland China. However, it is common for Western practitioners to use granules that are made in Taiwan, and the Taiwanese concept of formula combining is on the rise in the West. Several senior practitioners from Taiwan have begun training Westerners in the Taiwanese granule approach, and the widespread availability of whole formulas as well as single extracts has influenced the Western market. At present, Western countries do not have one single, well–defined approach to granules because multiple product styles exist on the market and relatively little academic training is available to guide new practitioners.

The remainder of this chapter will explore the major trends in granule dosage. First, single–dose sachets will be discussed. Single dose sachets are the most common form for granules in mainland China, and they are beginning to have a presence in the Western market. Next, dosage with loose granules of fixed concentration ratios will be discussed. These products and styles represent an important niche in the West.

Finally, this chapter will look at the Taiwanese method of dosing granules, as well as similar Western methods of determining dosage based on a total daily target dose. This latter approach is common for granules that have variable concentration ratios.

Method One: Using single–dose sachets

Concentration ratios express the relationship of the finished granule product to the raw herbs that went into it. Using concentration ratios to calculate dosage is common in regions that do not have a long history of granule use, such as mainland China and the U.S.. Practitioners accustomed to using raw herbs often use granules to replicate their typical raw herb dose weights, so they take the concentration ratio of the powder and use it to estimate how much powder is needed to approximate a given dose of raw herbs.

At the time of this writing, the challenge of dosage is compounded by the widespread lack of transparent labeling in the industry. Many suppliers do not provide data on concentration ratios, so estimating the desired dosage for a given case can be a challenge. As mentioned previously, the concentration ratios of products can vary significantly depending on the production method and the excipients used. For the sake of simplicity, this discussion on using sachets will focus on products with known, clearly stated concentration ratios.

The following dosage examples come from real products in mainland China, but will be presented without any identifying information as to the manufacturer. These examples have been randomly selected to illustrate the range of concentration ratios on the market and the different dosing strategies that apply.

Small sachets of granules are convenient for users that base dosage on raw herb weights. Typically, each sachet contains an average daily dose of a single medicinal, and one sachet is given per day of the prescription. The whole formula is made by combining 6–20 sachets or so, which are opened and mixed together in hot water as they are used.

This method is used in contradistinction to the method of mixing loose granules together. Loose granules often have a given concentration ratio (such as 5:1), and this ratio is used to calculate the dosage rather than using a single–dose sachet.

The main advantage of using single–dose sachets is that the powder does not need to be weighed, so the process of calculating dosage and filling the order is easy. Practitioners usually give one packet of each medicinal indicated, which delivers an average daily dose for each medicinal. A few items, such as Gan Cao (Glycyrrhizae Radix), are packaged in small doses of three grams to accommodate low doses; multiple sachets are simply given if six or nine grams are needed.

Another advantage of single–dose sachets lies in the ability to remove individual items if side effects appear. If a compound formula of ten medicinals is given and the patient experiences side effects, it is easy to remove one or two medicinals from the prescription because the granules remain in individual sachets.

On the downside, sachets can be a nuisance because many individual packets must be opened and mixed together for each dose. This generates a significant amount of packaging waste, and some users do not like having to open a dozen little packets with each dose. Another disadvantage of single–dose sachets is the fact that the herbs cannot be given in varying doses with ease; this is a nuisance for practitioners that wish to prescribe a daily dose of a given herb at a different quantity than the prepackaged, standard dose supplied.

On the next page are some examples of the concentration ratios and standard dosages found in sachet products. One sachet contains:

Medicinal with its standard granule dose and corresponding raw medicinal equivalent	Concentration Ratio
Dang Shen (Codonopsis Radix) 3.0g extract= 10 grams crude medicinal	3.33:1
Sha Shen (Glehniae Radix) 2.0g extract=10 grams crude medicinal	5:1
Dan Shen (Salviae Miltiorrhizae Radix) 2.0g extract=10 grams crude medicinal	5:1
San Qi (Notoginseng Radix) 3.0g = 3.0g (not concentrated)	1:1
Gan Cao (Glycyrrhizae Radix) 0.5g extract=3 grams crude medicinal	6:1
Ban Xia (Pinelliae Rhizoma) 0.5g extract=6 grams crude medicinal	12:1
Huang Qi (Astragali Radix) 1.5g extract=10 grams crude medicinal	6.66:1
Tu Fu Ling (Smilacis Glabrae Rhizoma) 1.0g extract=15 grams crude medicinal	15:1
San Leng (Sparganii Rhizoma) 0.5g extract= 10 grams crude medicinal	20:1
Cang Zhu (Atractylodis Rhizoma) 3g extract= 10 grams crude medicinal	3.33:1
Bai Zhu (Atractylodis Macrocephalae Rhizoma) 3g extract=10 grams crude medicinal	3.33:1
Chi Shao (Paeoniae Radix Rubra) 1.5g extract= 10 grams crude medicinal	6.66:1
Bai Shao (Paeoniae Radix Alba) 1g extract= 10 grams crude medicinal	10:1
Zhe Bei Mu (Fritillariae Thunbergii Bulbus) 1g extract=10 grams crude medicinal	10:1

From the previous example, we can clearly see that there is significant variation in the concentration ratios of the sachet products. However, each sachet contains a fairly even, average–strength dose, making the sachet delivery method fairly easy to use. Regardless of the precise concentration ratio or the brand chosen, each sachet has the granule equivalent of a standard dose of raw medicinals.

To understand the variations in concentration ratios on the market, it is interesting to compare the concentration ratios from one brand to the next. The main suppliers of granule sachets in mainland China use similar technology and excipients, but nonetheless there are still differences in the maximum concentrations attained from one brand to the next. The table below compares the same granule list above, but from two separate suppliers.

Medicinal	Concentration Ratio (Brand A)	Concentration Ratio (Brand B)
Dang Shen	3.33:1	3.3:1
Sha Shen	5:1	7.7:1
Dan Shen	5:1	5.6:1
San Qi	1:1	1:1
Gan Cao	6:1	6:1
Ban Xia	12:1	5:1
Huang Qi	6.66:1	5:1
Tu Fu Ling	15:1	7.5:1
San Leng	20:1	14.3:1
Cang Zhu	3.33:1	4.5:1
Bai Zhu	3.33:1	3.3:1
Chi Shao	6.66:1	5:1
Bai Shao	10:1	10:1
Zhe Bei Mu	10:1	5:1

The similarities and differences between these two products reveal that concentration ratios can be variable, even within similar products and manufacturing styles. There is a general similarity in the concentration ratios seen above, so one can see general trends. For example, San Leng is a very heavy, fibrous and dense root that naturally yields a high concentration ratio, whereas Dang Shen has a low concentration ratio because it is a moist, sticky root with much more water–soluble material.

When using granules in single–dose sachet packets, the concentration ratio does not matter much, because each sachet has the equivalent of one average day's dose. Therefore, a simple formula like Liu Jun Zi Tang (Six Gentlemen Decoction) could be mixed from single sachets as follows:

Medicinal	Decoction Dose (raw)	Granule Weight per sachet	Concentration Ratio	Number of Sachets
Bai Zhu (Atractylodis Macro-cephalae Rhizoma)	10g	3g	3.33:1	1
Fu Ling (Poria)	10g	0.5g	20:1	1
Ren Shen (Ginseng Radix)	5g	1.2g	4.2:1	1
Gan Cao (Glycyrrhizae Radix)	6g	0.5g	6:1	2
Chen Pi (Citri Reticulatae Pericarpium)	6g	1g	6:1	1
Ban Xia (Pinelliae Rhzoma)	10g	2g	5:1	1

In the above example, dosage with sachets is very easy. The formula is small and the dosage is very standard, so it is easy to fill the prescription and one can use an even number of sachets. For all items except Gan Cao (Glycyrrhizae Radix), only a single sachet is required.

Overall, granule sachets are particularly convenient for taking whole, unmodified formulas, especially when the whole formula is available in a single sachet. However, despite the general convenience of sachets, many practitioners prefer loose granules when mixing custom formulas because the dosage can be controlled more precisely. In the example above, the number of sachets is perfectly matched to the prescription, but any variation in the dosage of the medicinals listed above would cause the prescription to be less convenient in sachet form.

As a result of the fixed dose weights and the relatively high amount of waste generated by single–medicinal sachets, many consumers prefer granules that are packaged in loose bottles. Single–dose sachets do not expose the granule powder to air, so they can generally reach higher concentrations than granules that are packaged loose in bottles. When granules are packaged in 100–200 gram bottles, they usually require additional excipients so that the powder doesn't clump together upon exposure to air.

By adding excipients in different amounts, a manufacturer can achieve even concentration ratios in most products. The vast majority of medicinals can be produced at a 5:1 concentration, so 5:1 is the most common concentration ratio seen on most granule products coming out of mainland China.

Loose granule products at a standard 5:1 concentration stand in contradistinction to the single–dose sachets, which tend to vary from item to item in their concentration ratio. Consistent 5:1 loose granules are also slightly different than the typical granule products made in Taiwan. The Taiwanese granules also often reach 5:1, but they tend to vary significantly in their concentration ratio from product to product.

Dosing Granules with a 5:1 Concentration Ratio

Products that have an even 5:1 concentration ratio are very easy to use, because the dosage can be easily calculated by simple division. If a raw formula calls for 10 grams of a given medicinal, two grams of the granule extract can be used.

When using 5:1 concentrates, many practitioners simply dose the granules at about 0.5–3.0 grams per medicinal per day. Usually, the total daily target dose for a compound formula will be about 12–20 grams, with about 12–15 grams per day being fairly typical.

Fifteen grams of a 5:1 granule powder is equivalent to 75 grams of raw herbs, which is somewhat moderate for a raw herbal formula, as decoctions are commonly made with over 100 grams of raw herbs. However, there is a general consensus that the dosage can be reduced slightly from the equivalent raw herb dosage because the granule extraction process is more efficient than a home decoction. Thus, if 100 grams of raw herbs would be given to a particular patient as a home decoction, it would not be unreasonable to give 15 grams of 5:1 granules, which would equate to about 75 grams of raw herbs.

There is strong anecdotal support for the idea that granule doses can be reduced slightly from their precise raw herb equivalent. Many individual practitioners report that the results are satisfactory when using 12–18 grams of granules per day, which is mathematically a bit less than the same practitioners use in home decoctions (roughly equivalent to 60–90g/day instead of 80–150g/day). Additionally, research has begun to draw conclusions that support this clinical observation. One study demonstrated the increased efficiency of pressurized extraction techniques on constituents such as alkaloids and flavonoids, and at least one large–scale Chinese clinical trial has supported the idea that slight reductions in dosage may be appropriate when using granules.

To mix a prescription with 5:1 single medicinal extracts, simply write the prescription normally, with the standard raw decoction doses as a guide. Divide the raw doses by five to determine the granule dosage. Many practitioners round down, or use slightly less than the exact equivalent dose for the reasons listed above. However, the basic method still applies. Consider the following example:

Medicinal	Decoction Dose (raw)	Concentration Ratio	Granule Weight
Suan Zao Ren (Ziziphi Spinosi Semen)	12g	5:1	2.5g
Fu Ling (Poria)	10g	5:1	2.0g
Chuan Xiong (Chuanxiong Rhizoma)	5g	5:1	1.0g
Zhi Mu (Anemarrhenae Rhizoma)	8g	5:1	1.5g
Gan Cao (Glycyrrhizae Radix)	3g	5:1	0.5g
Ye Jiao Teng (Polygoni Multiflori Caulis)	15g	5:1	3.0g
He Huan Pi (Albizziae Cortex)	12g	5:1	2.5g
Bai Zi Ren (Platycladi Semen)	10g	5:1	2.0g
Bai Shao (Paeoniae Radix Alba)	10g	5:1	2.0g
Total	85g		17.0g

In the above example, the formula is not large and the doses could probably be reduced slightly. To prepare a supply of the formula above, the doses in the "granule weight" column can simply be multiplied by the number of days desired. This method is very straightforward and commonly used.

The only weakness with this method lies in its reliance on the availability of products with even 5:1 concentration ratios across the board. Only a few suppliers produce entire lines of 5:1 extracts, and there are a few individual items that cannot reach 5:1 concentrations. Often, the exceptions are not clearly labeled or recognized, so practitioners mistakenly assume that 100% of a given product line consists of 5:1 extracts.

As we see in the examples above, even the products produced in sachets do not always achieve 5:1 concentrations. Medicinals such as Dang Gui (Angelicae Sinensis Radix), Gou Qi Zi (Lycii Fructus), and Da Zao (Jujubae Fructus) are sticky and rich in water–soluble constituents, so they are hard to concentrate at levels higher than 3:1. Gelatins and some expensive products such as Chen Xiang (Aquilariae Lignum Resinatum) and Ge Jie (Gecko) are generally 1:1 powders rather than concentrated extracts. Practitioners must be mindful of these exceptions so that they can adjust doses accordingly.

Ideally, suppliers should provide full disclosure on the concentration ratio of each product. It is common for suppliers of products with significantly variable concentrations to claim that their products are generally 5:1, even when they are not. Likewise, some suppliers that specialize in 5:1 products tend to say that all of their products are 5:1, and often gloss over the fact that 10% or so are not truly 5:1.

Below is a partial list of products that are commonly sold in concentrations under 5:1. These items often need to be assessed individually, as their concentration ratios tend to vary from one supplier to the next.

Dang Shen	Codonopsis Radix
Da Zao	Jujubae Fructus
Tian Dong	Asparagi Radix
Shan Zha	Crataegi Fructus
Shan Zhu Yu	Corni Fructus
Shan Yao	Dioscoreae Rhizoma
Ba Ji Tian	Morindae Officinalis Radix

Dang Gui	Angelicae Sinensis Radix
Gou Qi Zi	Lycii Fructus
Shu Di Huang	Rehmanniae Radix Praeparata
Xuan Shen	Scrophulariae Radix
Sheng Di Huang	Rehmanniae Radix
Rou Cong Rong	Cistanches Herba
Mai Dong	Ophiopogonis Radix
Long Yan Rou	Longan Arillus
Chen Xiang	Aquilariae Lignum Resinatum
E Jiao	Asini Corii Colla
Ge Jie	Gecko
Shui Zhi	Hirudo
Zhu Sha	Cinnabaris
Chuan Bei Mu	Fritillariae Cirrhosae Bulbus
Xi Yang Shen	Panacis Quinquefolii Radix
San Qi	Notoginseng Radix
Qing Dai	Indigo Naturalis
Zi He Che	Hominis Placenta
Tan Xiang	Santali Albi Lignum
Lu Hui	Aloe
Bai Bu	Stemonae Radix

In some markets, such as Canada and Taiwan, information on concentration ratios is part of the standard labeling and is required by law. However, the U.S. has no such labeling requirement, so practitioners must ask their vendors about any questions on concentration ratios that arise. There is more to granules than concentration ratios, and there are many excellent suppliers that produce granules with variable concentration ratios. Practitioners should look beyond concentration ratios alone, but ideally concentration ratios should be clearly labeled so that guesswork is not required.

Dosing 3:1, 6:1, and 9:1 granule products

Until relatively recently, most granule products on the market coming from mainland China have been sold in either single–dose sachets or as 5:1 extracts. Both of these methods are effective, but each offers distinct advantages and disadvantages.

The sachets have an advantage in that they require minimal filler and tend to be accurately labeled with regard to their raw herb equivalent. However, sachets produce more waste and offer less flexibility with dosage. By contrast, the loose 5:1 extracts are easier to use at any dosage desired, and a single bottle of mixed loose granules can contain a week's worth of a given prescription. The only major disadvantage of the 5:1 method is the fact that items with a low natural concentration ratio cannot easily reach 5:1, and items with a naturally high concentration ratio must be diluted down to 5:1.

In an effort to minimize excipients and offer even potency, some suppliers have recently begun producing granules at three tiers of concentration ratios: 3:1, 6:1, and 9:1. A three–tiered approach is a very innovative way to solve the issue of varied concentration ratios. This method allows dosage to be easily calculated based on a standard raw decoction prescription, and it minimizes unnecessary fillers by allowing some products to be sold at a higher concentration.

In this method, items that can naturally achieve high concentration ratios are made to an even 9:1 concentration, reducing the need for excipients (if the product is diluted to 5:1, it would require nearly 40% more excipient). Items that can achieve 6:1 concentrations form the middle tier. Finally, the few substances that are sticky and exceptionally rich in water–soluble constituents are concentrated to 3:1.

Concentration ratios of 3:1, 6:1, and 9:1 are convenient because many practitioners dose their raw herbs in multiples of three. It is common to see raw herb prescriptions that contain 3g, 6g, 9g, 12g, 15g, or 30g of a given medicinal, and the three–tiered concentration ratio can be easily used to convert such decoction weights into a granule equivalent. Consider the following example:

Medicinal	Decoction Dose (raw)	Concentration Ratio	Granule Weight
Dang Gui (Angelicae Sinensis Radix)	9g	3:1	3.0g
Chi Shao (Paeoniae Radix Rubra)	9g	6:1	1.5g
Chuan Xiong (Chuanxiong Rhizoma)	6g	6:1	1.0g
Shu Di Huang (Rehmanniae Radix Praeparata)	12g	3:1	4.0g
Tao Ren (Persicae Semen)	9g	9:1	1.0g
Hong Hua (Carthami Flos Sichuanensis)	9g	6:1	1.5g
Chai Hu (Bupleuri Radix)	6g	6:1	1.0g
Bai Shao (Paeoniae Radix Alba)	12g	6:1	2.0g
Gan Cao (Glycyrrhizae Radix)	3g	6:1	0.5g
Total	75g		15.5g

In the example above, very accurate dosing is obtained. Compared to using loose granules that vary in concentration from product to product, the three–tiered approach makes calculation based on raw decoction doses very simple. By producing some products at 3:1, some at 6:1, and some at 9:1, there is less pressure to force individual herbs to a concentration ratio that is unnaturally high or unnaturally low. This allows for transparency in labeling and relatively low use of excipients.

Dosing styles in Taiwan

In Taiwan, granules have been used extensively because they are the only herbal products that are covered by the national health insurance system. While the insurance system limits the maximum dose that a doctor can prescribe, the inclusion of granules into the national insurance system has stimulated tremendous research and experience in the use of granules. There is nowhere in the world that uses granules more frequently than Taiwan, so the Taiwanese experience is invaluable in assessing the granule field.

Granule prescriptions in Taiwan are generally created by combining multiple base formulas together. In addition to starting with whole formulas, Taiwanese doctors commonly add single medicinal extracts when customizing the prescription. This practice of combining base formulas with single–herb additions is one of the most distinctive features of Chinese medicine in Taiwan.

The vast majority of practitioners in Taiwan believe that combining whole granule formulas that were cooked together is superior to using single extracts to build a formula from scratch. In truth, this viewpoint is so pervasive that few doctors in Taiwan have tried prescribing granules any other way. While it is impossible to assess whether the Taiwanese method objectively yields superior results, the efficacy of their method has been well–demonstrated in millions of patient visits.

In Taiwan, it is common for the clinic to mix a granule prescription and dispense it in small plastic bags. The plastic bags are formed by a machine that divides the powder into specified doses, eliminating the need for the patient to measure the powder with a spoon. The prescription is recorded in the patient's digital file, and a printout is usually included with the prescription from the pharmacy.

According to research conducted by Dr. Chang Hsien–Cheh of China Medical University in Taiwan, over 60 million patient visits that used granules were recorded by Taiwan's National Health Insurance system during 2004 and 2005. During this two–year time period, over 4,000 Chinese medical doctors prescribed nearly 2.7 million kilograms of granule extracts. This represents the most complete digital database of granule therapy in the world.

The national insurance system in Taiwan pays for up to six grams of granules per dose. The typical six–gram dose is usually given three times per day, for a total of 18g of concentrated extract powder per day. The precise extraction ratios for each product are clearly stated on the granule labels in Taiwan. However, most doctors there think less in terms of calculating extraction ratios and replicating raw herb doses by weight, and focus more on the ratio of herbs and formulas within the daily target dose of 18g/day.

The dosage used by most doctors in Taiwan tends to fluctuate between 12–18 grams/day, with 18 grams being the most common for adults. Taiwan's insurance system uses a digital chip embedded in an ID card that is linked to the patient's chart. The computer system that hospitals and clinics use with the insurance card does not allow the dosage of granules to exceed six grams per dose, so most practitioners think about granule dosage within the context of a six–gram single dose. The total dose that is entered is usually 4–6 grams, and each dose is given three times per day.

The dosage of granule prescriptions in Taiwan is generally calculated based on the relative proportions of a given medicinal or formula within the maximum six–gram dose. Many Taiwanese doctors have mastered a huge repertoire of formulas, so their prescriptions often contain classical formulas that may not be familiar to most Western practitioners.

Each six–gram dose tends to contain about 4–6 grams of formulas that treat the chief presenting pattern. For secondary patterns, whole formulas are commonly added in a dose range of 0.3–1.2 grams. Singles are often added at a dose of 0.1–1 gram TID (three times per day). The most common dose range seen for singles is about 0.3g TID, or about one gram per day for most items.

Below are some examples, taken from the author's observation of doctors at Chang Gung Memorial Hospital in Taiwan. All of these prescriptions come from senior practitioners. While the case notes provided are often not sufficient to illustrate the patient's full clinical picture, the dosage levels and complexity of the formulas illustrates the standard approach used in Taiwan.

Example One:

In the gynecology department, female patients would commonly come in for treatment for late menstruation. The doctor would typically administer a pregnancy test, and if the pregnancy test was negative, the following formula was fairly common:

> Xue Fu Zhu Yu Tang (House of Blood Stasis–Expelling Decoction) 3.5 g
>
> E Zhu (Curcumae Rhizoma) 0.3 g
>
> Ze Lan (Lycopi Herba) 0.3 g

This formula is very small, but it is relatively straightforward; 4.1 grams were given per dose, for a total of about 12.3 grams per day. If the above formula failed to bring on menstruation within a few days, a more customized formula would typically be indicated.

Example Two:

In another example, consider the following formula for a patient suffering from cough and sinus congestion:

> Xin Yi San (Officinal Magnolia Flower Powder) 2.0 g
>
> Cang Er Zi San (Xanthium Powder) 0.75 g
>
> Xiao Qing Long Tang (Minor Black Dragon Decoction) 0.3 g
>
> Ma Xing Gan Shi Tang (Ephedra, Apricot Kernel, Gypsum, and Licorice Decoction) 1.25 g
>
> E Bu Shi Cao (Centipedae Herba) 0.2 g
>
> Lu Lu Tong (Liquidambaris Fructus) 0.2 g
>
> Zao Jiao Ci (Gleditsiae Spina) 0.2 g

Here, 4.9 grams of granules were given three times per day, for a total of about 14.7 grams per day. Note the complex use of formulas in this prescription. Four whole formulas are prescribed simultaneously. The formulas together make up 4.3 grams, or about 88% of the total dose, but no single formula is used at a dose of over 2.0 grams. Combining as many as four formulas together is not uncommon in Taiwan, but many prescriptions do use fewer formulas than this.

Example Three:

Consider the following prescription, given to a 34 year–old female with peeling skin and blistering skin on her hands. She had a history of summerheat strike, a dry mouth with bitter taste, raised red papilla (cinnabar spots) on her tongue, white fur, insomnia, increased vaginal discharge, and slight constipation. She was prescribed:

Ba Wei Dai Xia Fang (Eight–Ingredient Discharge Formula) 1.2 g

Jing Fang Bai Du San (Schizonepeta and Saposhnikovia Toxin–Vanquishing Powder) 1.8 g

Di Fu Zi (Kochiae Fructus) 0.4 g

Cang Zhu (Atractylodis Rhizoma) 0.3 g

Sang Zhi (Mori Ramulus) 0.3 g

Bai Xian Pi (Dictamni Cortex) 0.5 g

Zi Cao (Arnebiae/Lithospermi Radix) 0.3 g

Pu Gong Ying (Taraxaci Herba) 0.3 g

Mai Men Dong (Ophiopogonis Radix) 0.3 g

This patient was given 5.4 grams of granules per dose, for a total of 16.2 grams per day. Her prescription contains two whole formulas and seven single medicinals.

Example Four:

The following prescription was given to a middle–aged male patient with chronic hepatitis. He exhibited pitting edema in the lower legs, and had a large, slightly red tongue with yellow fur.

Da Chai Hu Tang (Major Bupleurum Decoction) 1.5 g

Jiang Can (Bombyx Batryticatus) 0.3 g

Chan Tui (Cicadae Periostracum) 0.3 g

Lu Gen (Phragmitis Rhizoma) 0.3 g

Chi Shao (Paeoniae Radix Rubra) 0.3 g

Tao Ren (Persicae Semen) 0.3 g

Long Dan Xie Gan Tang (Gentian Liver–Draining Decoction) 2 g

Huang Lian (Coptidis Rhizoma) 0.3 g

Bai Shao (Paeoniae Radix Alba) 0.3 g

Bie Jia (Trionycis Carapax) 0.4 g

Here, the total dose was 6 g, given three times per day for a total of 18 g per day.

Example Five:

The following prescription was given to 42 year–old female patient with Sjogren's Syndrome, rheumatoid arthritis, and urticaria. She had swel– ling and pain at her knuckles and had poor sleep, thick slimy tongue fur and a dark tongue with stasis and a red tip. She also suffered from recent insomnia.

Shu Jing Huo Xue Tang (Channel–Coursing Blood–Quickening Decoction) 1.5 g

Gan Lu Yin (Sweet Dew Beverage) 1.5 g

Long Dan Xie Gan Tang (Gentian Liver–Draining Decoction) 1.5 g

Mu Dan Pi (Moutan Cortex) 0.5 g

Yi Yi Ren (Coicis Semen) 0.4 g

Chi Shao (Paeoniae Radix Rubra) 0.3 g

Mu Gua (Chaenomelis Fructus) 0.3 g

This prescription was prescribed at a total dose of 6.0 grams, three times per day (18 g/day). It contains three formulas in even proportions.

Example Six:

The following prescription was given to a 35 year–old female patient with lupus (SLE), presenting with a rash from her feet up to her calves. She had a thin red tongue with a thin coat that was peeled at the edges. She reported no current pain or itching, and had a thin rough pulse. She experiences dry lips and dry throat.

Gan Lu Yin (Sweet Dew Beverage) 1.5 g

Long Dan Xie Gan Tang (Gentian Liver–Draining Decoction) 1.5 g

Yin Qiao San (Lonicera and Forsythia Powder) 1.5 g

Mu Dan Pi (Moutan Cortex) 0.3 g

Bai Shao (Paeoniae Radix Alba) 0.3 g

Yi Yi Ren (Coicis Semen) 0.3 g

Sang Bai Pi (Mori Cortex) 0.3 g

Here, 5.9 grams of granules were prescribed three times per day, for a total of 17.7 grams per day.

Example Seven:

The following prescription was given to a 53 year–old female with tinnitus, dizziness, and poor sleep. She gets a dry mouth with a bitter taste, anxiety, and a history of pain and swelling in her knee, along with frequent crying.

Mu Gua (Chaenomelis Fructus) 0.4 g

Zhi Bai Di Huang Wan (Anemarrhena, Phellodendron, and Rehmannia Pill) 1.4 g

Suan Zao Ren Tang (Spiny Jujube Decoction) 1.2 g

San Qi (Notoginseng Radix) 0.4 g

Tian Ma Gou Teng Yin (Gastrodia and Uncaria Beverage) 1.4 g

Dang Gui (Angelicae Sinensis Radix) 0.4 g

Bai Shao (Paeoniae Radix Alba) 0.4 g

Tian Men Dong (Asparagi Radix) 0.4 g

This patient was prescribed 6.0 grams of granules three times per day, for a total of 18 grams per day.

Example Eight:

A young female child presented with common cold characterized by cough and wheezing with little phlegm. She had a red tongue and slightly red eyes.

Ma Xing Gan Shi Tang (Ephedra, Apricot Kernel, Licorice, and Gypsum Decoction) 0.6 g

Ding Chuan Tang (Panting–Stabilizing Decoction) 1.2 g

Pi Pa Ye (Eriobotryae Folium) 0.2 g

This formula illustrates granule dosage for a child. Here, we see that 2.0 grams are given per dose, for a total of only 6 grams per day. The use of small doses is common in children. Children often receive dosage at about 1/3 to 1/2 of the standard adult dosage, and the dosage can be further reduced for patients that are very young.

Example Nine:

The following prescription was given to a patient that suffers from infertility and endometriosis. She had just received a hormonal check and all the results came back within normal limits. She had a pale tongue with cold hands, and her pattern presented with signs of kidney yang vacuity and liver depression.

Jia Wei Xiao Yao San (Supplemented Free Wanderer Powder) 3.0g

You Gui Wan (Right–Restoring Pill) 2.5 g

Yin Yang Huo (Epimedii Herba) 0.5 g

Here, 6.0 grams were given three times per day, for a total of 18 grams per day. Note the use of two compound formulas with only a single addition.

Example Ten:

The patient was an 11 year–old male with allergic rhinitis. He has experienced sneezing, clear nasal discharge, and sinus congestion for several years. These symptoms are particularly prevalent upon awakening. Postnasal drip and cough are occasionally noted, along with frequent throat clearing. He has no history of food allergies or asthma, although blood tests indicate an allergic response to eggs, shrimp, and mites. He was diagnosed with lung and spleen qi vacuity.

Xiao Qing Long Tang (Minor Green–Blue Dragon Decoction) 0.4 g

Xin Yi San (Officinal Magnolia Flower Powder) 2.8 g

Xiang Sha Liu Jun Zi Tang (Costusroot and Amomum Six Gentlemen Decoction) 0.4 g

Here, we see the use of granules at a dose of 3.6 grams, given three times per day (13.2 grams total). This dose range is somewhat lower than the typical adult dose, but it is consistent for a child of eleven years of age. This formula relies on Xin Yi San to open the nose, complemented by a small amount of Xiao Qing Long Tang to warm cold–rheum and eliminate wind–cold. Xiang Sha Liu Jun Zi Tang is used to support the spleen to treat the root problem of phlegm.

Overall, Taiwan uses a very distinctive and innovative approach to granules. Doctors in Taiwan have a tremendous degree of experience with granules, but their approach has not been adequately studied and implemented outside of Taiwan.

Even within Taiwan, there are not any books or training courses that truly provide comprehensive training in the local granule approach. Doctors tend to imitate their teachers, and forty years of granule use in Taiwan has slowly caused a distinctive style to emerge. Taiwan has a number of excellent granule suppliers and hundreds of clinical experts, so the global impact of Taiwan on the granule field cannot be underestimated.

The Taiwanese method of formula combining is truly a new development in Chinese medicine, and Taiwan's digital system is unique in its ability to gather statistical data and evidence–based results derived from the local granule approach. As time goes on, hopefully our community will see more and more literature on Taiwan's approach to granules and formula combining.

Western Trends in Granule Dosage

In the West, it is common for practitioners to utilize a hybrid system of granule dosage that has characteristics of both the mainland and Taiwanese approach. At present, relatively little training is available for Western practitioners, and a variety of competing messages on dosage exists in the West.

Unfortunately, many practitioners in the West have had little exposure to the granule dosing trends in Asia. Compounding this problem, relatively few products provide information on their concentration ratios when they are labeled for Western markets such as the U.S.. At the time of this writing, most granule labels in the U.S. do not provide transparency on concentrations or clear instructions for use, which leads many practitioners with no source of information on dosage other than the generic advice of the vendors themselves.

Asking vendors for advice on dosage has a number of limitations. If the vendors recommend high doses, they fear that customers will regard their product as less potent. Furthermore, the vendors cannot reliably trust the skill of the practitioner, so they may be hesitant to recommend high doses. Finally, the vendor may personally believe that high doses are superior, but their products may be labeled with an artificially low dosage recommendation; this leaves the vendor in an awkward situation because they do not want to contradict their marketing materials yet they may sincerely want to offer better information on dosage. Consequently, vendors are not an ideal source of information on dosage.

U.S. FDA law requires manufacturers to list one specific dose on the label; a general range is not permitted. However, the dosage that is specified on the bottle often has little to do with clinical reality. It is common for suppliers to list a very low dose on the bottle, because this practice makes the bottle appear to contain more servings and thus offer better value. Additionally, recommending a low dose on the bottle reduces the likelihood of adverse effects and litigation for the manufacturer. These factors provide manufacturers with a strong incentive to state a very conservative dose on the label.

One often hears dramatically different advice from manufacturers on issues of dosage. For example, some suppliers routinely advise practitioners to use 6 grams of granules per day, while others advise 6–12 grams per day or 12–18 grams per day. In many instances, single extracts are labeled with one generic dose that is recommended for all medicinals. Confounding this problem, one major textbook on herbal formulas states that 10 grams is the standard daily dose in Taiwan, which differs significantly from this author's experience of 12–18 grams being the standard dose range in Taiwan.

Given that many suppliers conceal information on concentration ratios and offer dramatically different advice on dosage, it is not surprising that dosage is a confusing issue for many Western granule users. Ideally, schools would be a good place for education on granule dosage, but most schools currently lack training on this subject. In fact, many schools train students to use a mathematical system of calculating granule doses without any regard to whether the mathematical equation has any intrinsic validity for the granules that are actually being used.

For example, it is common for student clinics in the U.S. to prescribe granule doses based on a fixed concentration ratio. In such a model, students compose a raw decoction prescription and then use division to determine the appropriate granule dose. While this method is effective for products that have a consistent concentration ratio, it is largely useless for items where the concentration ratio is not stated or consistent.

All too often, school clinics teach students to prescribe granules as though they were at a 5:1 concentration, without ever investigating whether the products used are actually 5:1. In fact, the most common products on the market in the U.S. come from Taiwan, where the concentration ratios generally range from 3:1–5:1. This makes a mathematical equation based on 5:1 nonsensical.

The easiest way to calculate granule dosage is to think about the target dose that is desired, and then dose the ingredients within the formula based on their relative importance and potency. Large formulas will tend to require higher doses, while small formulas can get by with lower doses. Additionally, the dosing strategy changes slightly depending on whether single extracts or compound formulas are used.

Dosing Formulas Made From Singles

In general, the total adult granule dosage should be between 10–18 grams per day. For severe and acute conditions, 15–25 grams per day or more can be used. For children, the dosage often ranges from 3–10 grams per day. For the sake of simplicity, let us use an example based on an average patient that is being prescribed 10–18 grams per day.

First, consider the total amount that is going to be prescribed per day. If prescribing a formula with 15–18 ingredients, the total dose should be closer to 18 grams per day. If only 5–12 ingredients are used, a dosage of 10–18 grams is probably sufficient. If the case is mild or the patient is weak, the dosage should be on the low side. If the case is severe or the patient is large and robust, the dosage should be on the high side. As a rule of thumb, multiplying the number of ingredients by 1.5 should give a reasonable total daily dose.

Next, consider how many medicinals are in the prescription. If 18 grams will be prescribed and 12 ingredients are used, the average dose of each medicinal will be about 1.5 grams.

In any given formula, some items will be used at higher doses than others. Medicinals that are potent by weight or extreme in nature should be given at low doses, generally 0.3–1.5 grams per day. Examples include items such as Rou Gui (Cinnamomi Cortex), Ren Shen (Ginseng Radix), Fu Zi (Aconiti Radix Lateralis Praeparata), Sha Ren (Amomi Fructus), Chai Hu (Bupleuri Radix), and Wu Zhu Yu (Evodiae Fructus).

By contrast, medicinals that have a balanced nature and a relatively high standard dose in raw decoctions should be used at higher doses, typically 1–3 grams per day. Examples include items like Shu Di Huang (Rehmanniae Radix Praeparata), Shan Yao (Dioscoreae Rhizoma), Yi Yi Ren (Coicis Semen), Mu Li (Ostreae Concha), and Yu Zhu (Polygonati Odorati Rhizoma).

Items that have a moderate, mid–range dosage in decoctions are often used at a dose of 1–2 grams per day. Such items include Dang Gui (Angelicae Sinensis Radix), Bai Zhu (Atractylodis Macrocephalae Rhizoma), Bai Shao (Paeoniae Radix Alba), Ba Ji Tian (Morindae Officinalis Radix), etc.

Some items are used at different dosages for different purposes. For example, Chai Hu (Bupleuri Radix) is often used in low doses to raise yang in formulas such as Bu Zhong Yi Qi Tang (Center–Supplementing Qi–Boosting Decoction). In such applications, 0.3–0.8 grams of granule Chai Hu is generally sufficient. If Chai Hu is instead used to course the liver qi, slightly larger granule doses are typical, such as 0.5–1.5 grams. For treating lesser yang disease, even higher quantities would be called for, such as 1.5–3.0 grams. Similarly, Gan Cao (Glycyrrhizae Radix) is generally used at a low dose as a courier to harmonize a formula (0.5–1.0 grams), but it can be used in high doses (2–3 grams) as a sovereign medicinal in a formula such as Zhi Gan Cao Tang (Honey–Fried Licorice Decoction).

Consider the following examples. In the first example, a small formula with only 8 ingredients is used. In this example, the daily target dose will be around 12 grams.

Medicinal	Granule Dose	Notes	Typical Raw Dose
Ren Shen (Ginseng Radix)	1.2g	Potent by weight	3–10g
Fu Ling (Poria)	2.5g	Mild by weight	6–15g
Chen Pi (Citri Reticulatae Pericarpium)	1.0g	Potent by weight	3–10g
Gan Jiang (Zingiberis Rhizoma)	1.0g	Potent by weight	3–10g
Gan Cao (Glycyrrhizae Radix)	0.5g	Used to harmonize	3–6g
Bai Zhu (Atractylodis Macrocephalae Rhizoma)	1.8g	Moderate	3–15g
Huang Qi (Astragali Radix)	2.5g	Mild by weight	10–30g
Ban Xia (Pinelliae Rhizoma)	1.5g	Moderate	6–12g
Total	12g		

Consider the example below, with a larger formula of 12 ingredients. Here, the total daily target dose will be about 18 grams.

Medicinal	Granule Dose	Notes	Typical Raw Dose
Ren Shen (Ginseng Radix)	2.5g	Mild by weight	6–15g
Fu Ling (Poria)	1.2g	Moderate	6–15g
Bai Shao (Paeoniae Radix Alba)	1.5g	Moderate	6–15g
Zhi Gan Cao (Glycyrrhizae Radix Praeparata)	0.5g	Used to harmonize	3–6g
Bai Zhu (Atractylodis Macrocephalae Rhizoma)	1.5g	Moderate	3–15g
Shu Di Huang (Rehmanniae Radix Praeparata)	2.8g	Mild by weight	10–30g
Suan Zao Ren (Ziziphi Spinosi Semen)	1.5g	Moderate	6–15g
Ye Jiao Teng (Polygoni Multiflori Caulis)	2.0g	Mild by weight	10–30g
Chai Hu (Bupleuri Radix)	1.0g	Potent by weight	3–10g
Xiang Fu (Cyperi Rhizoma)	1.5g	Moderate	6–12g
Chuan Xiong (Chuanxiong Rhizoma)	1.0g	Potent by weight	3–12g
Total	18g		

In a larger formula such as this one, there are many factors to pay attention to. The medicinals should always be in proportion to the patient's presentation. For example, if blood vacuity is prominent, the relative doses of medicinals such as Shu Di Huang, Bai Shao, and Dang Gui should be relatively high. Within those three, Shu Di Huang will tend to be the highest because its raw dose standard is the highest. Bai Shao and Dang Gui can be used at similar dose ranges, but Dang Gui is somewhat prone to producing side–effects such as diarrhea if its dosage is too high.

The fundamental nature of each medicinal should always be taken into account. Shu Di Huang is rich and potentially stagnating, so its dosage should not be excessive in patients that are prone to dampness and diarrhea. Chuan Xiong and Chai Hu are relatively dry medicinals, so their dosage should not be too high for most cases. Fu Ling and Ye Jiao Teng are relatively weak medicinals by weight, so their dosage should be relatively high. Zhi Gan Cao is used to harmonize here, so its dosage should be low. Medicinals such as Xiang Fu, Bai Shao, and Bai Zhu are here being used at a moderate dosage, not too high and not too low.

Dosage When Combining Formulas

If one is starting with base formulas, the dosing strategy changes slightly. Again, the total daily target dose will tend to be about 12–18 grams for the final prescription, but the quantities of each item within the formula will tend to be higher since whole formulas are used instead of single extracts.

When combining several formulas together that have similar principles, the dosage of both formulas can be reduced. For example, if Liu Jun Zi Tang (Six Gentlemen Decoction) and Bu Zhong Yi Qi Tang (Center–Supplementing Qi–Boosting Decoction) were used together, the dosage of each one could be reduced.

If one formula treats the main pattern and it is combined with a second formula that addresses a specific symptom or an auxiliary pattern, the main formula should be used at a dose of 8–12 grams and the auxiliary formula for the secondary pattern or symptom should be used at a dose of 1–6 grams. For example, to treat constipation due to liver depression, 12 grams of Xiao Yao San (Free Wanderer Powder) could be used with

4–6 grams of Ma Zi Ren Wan (Cannabis Seed Pill). In this instance, Xiao Yao San would be used to treat the root pattern of liver depression, while Ma Zi Ren Wan would be added to provide symptomatic relief for the constipation.

If two formulas are used with equal emphasis, they should have roughly similar doses, especially if they have a comparable number of ingredients. For example, the formula Si Ni San (Counterflow Cold Powder) is commonly combined with the formula Tong Xie Yao Fang (Painful Diarrhea Formula) to treat diarrhea and pain due to a wood–earth disharmony. Both of these formulas have the same number of ingredients and both may be equally important for the condition, so the dose of each one could be 6–8 grams.

If three or more formulas are used together, the dosage of each formula tends to be lower than it would be if only one base formula was used. If three or more formulas are combined, the dosage of each formula is often only 2–6 grams.

When using a whole formula as though it were a single medicinal addition, the dosage can be quite low. A single medicinal addition is usually added at a dose of 0.5–3.0 grams per day, and this same dose range could be used for a whole formula. For example, if one added Huang Lian Jie Du Tang (Coptis Toxin–Resolving Decoction) to a formula instead of adding a single medicinal such as Huang Lian (Coptidis Rhizoma), the whole formula could be added at a low dose such as 0.5 grams.

Example One:

A patient presents with diarrhea that is accompanied by tenesmus and pain. Upon examination, the patient is diagnosed with a wood–earth disharmony complicated by damp–heat. The following prescription is given:

> Si Ni San (Counterflow Cold Powder) 6 grams
>
> Tong Xie Yao Fang (Painful Diarrhea Formula) 6 grams
>
> Huang Lian (Coptidis Rhizoma) 1 gram
>
> Mu Xiang (Aucklandiae Radix) 1 gram

In this example, two compound formulas are used together, with two single medicinal additions. A total daily dose of 14 grams is used. Si Ni San and Tong Xie Yao Fang address wood–earth disharmony manifesting in painful diarrhea. Huang Lian and Mu Xiang are added here to eliminate tenesmus due to damp–heat.

Example Two:

A patient presents with constipation prior to menstruation. She experiences mood swings, irritability, painful menstruation, delayed menstruation, and breast distention. She is diagnosed with liver depression and mild blood stasis. She is prescribed the following formula:

> Jia Wei Xiao Yao San (Supplemented Free Wanderer Powder) 8 grams
>
> Tao He Cheng Qi Tang (Peach Kernel Qi–Infusing Decoction) 2 grams
>
> Qing Pi, 0.8 grams
>
> Yu Jin, 1.0 grams
>
> Xiang Fu, 1.2 grams

Here, the patient is given a combination of two formulas with three single additions. The principle formula, Jia Wei Xiao Yao San, addresses the liver depression and irritability that is central to her diagnosis. The secondary formula, Tao He Cheng Qi Tang, frees the stool and quickens the blood. Although Tao He Cheng Qi Tang contains Gui Zhi (Cinnamomi Ramulus) and is slightly warm, it is used at a relatively low dose here and its warm temperature is offset by the cool nature of Jia Wei Xiao Yao San. Qing Pi, Xiang Fu, and Yu Jin together strengthen the qi–moving nature of the formula and help to relieve the breast distention.

Conclusion

Dosage is a very important aspect of the clinical application of granules. In this chapter, we have seen several different therapeutic approaches presented. Each of these approaches has been extensively tested in clinic, and each method has its adherents. The use of granules is an emerging science, and it is essential to keep an open mind about the different strategies that are available.

All too often, practitioners view the issue of dosage with unnecessary rigidity. Some practitioners insist upon very strict mathematical calculations while others use broad estimates. Some practitioners dose their granules in a nearly identical fashion as they dose their decoctions, while others use granules in much lower dosages or use them with a totally different compounding style. At present, it is impossible to broadly assert the superiority of a single method because the landscape is too diverse and the various systems have not been extensively compared with one another in clinical trials.

The topic of granules is a fascinating subject precisely because it is largely unexplored in the academic world. Granules represent a multi-disciplinary field of research, and people with expertise in granules come from a variety of backgrounds. Some experts are chemists, some are clinicians, some are engineers, and some are entrepreneurs. Each expert has a particular viewpoint based on their own experience, but no one person has expertise in all the collective disciplines that affect granules.

Consequently, it is important to study widely and gain exposure to multiple styles and perspectives. At present, the world of granules is largely fragmented. For example, mainland China and Taiwan each have major experts and excellent factories, but both regions are largely unaware of the developments in their neighbor's backyard. Practitioners in both places broadly assert that the other region does it all wrong and boast that they alone have the correct approach. In truth, both sides make valid arguments and both regions have developed viable approaches that have proven to be clinically successful.

In many ways, the world of granules is influenced by the complex politics between mainland China and Taiwan. Invariably, if one travels regularly to both regions, one is stricken by the fact that there is significant regional prejudice on both sides of the water. There is generally insufficient academic exchange between the two regions, and their first real experience butting heads in the commercial world of granules is occurring for the first time right now, in overseas markets such as the U.S., Canada, and Singapore. If a practitioner doesn't understand the complex history between these two regions, it is easy to be blinded by one-sided arguments.

In fact, a similar issue exists between China, Korea, and Japan. The long–held cultural barriers and grudges in East Asian society influence regional perspectives on medicine, and all too often we see blanket criticisms of the medical practice of an entire region. Depending on where one happens to be, this prejudice will be targeted at a different group, but the fundamental issue is the same. If one has never experienced the strong regional attitudes that are common in East Asia, one may not grasp all the issues involved in comparing perspectives on something as innocent as granules.

The issues related to granule dosage are complex and multi–faceted. The field is new even in the Chinese world, and there are multiple perspectives to consider on many issues. Most people that gain exposure to the diverse landscape of methods used end up concluding that the situation with granule dosage is far from simple and has more than one right answer.

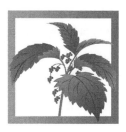

CHAPTER SIX

The Art of Formula Combining

The practice of combining whole formulas is a widespread new trend in the field of Chinese medicine. Formula combining is not an entirely new trend by any means, but the current widespread availability of prepared formulas has allowed the practice of formula combining to expand significantly.

The practice of formula combining is particularly prevalent with granule extracts, and formula combining is a fundamental feature of the basic method of granule use as practiced in Taiwan and Japan. Formula combining is comparatively less common in mainland China, where single herb extracts and raw herbs dominate the market. In the West, we use formula combining on a small scale with granule products and liquid concentrates, but most Western practitioners lack experience and training in the principles of formula combining.

Historically, we find many examples where a compound formula like Liu Yi San (Six to One Powder) was used as an addition to a whole formula. In the modern day, the availability of hundreds of pre–made granule formulas has greatly expanded the scope of formulas that can be easily combined.

Granule formulas are commonly built from mixing single–herb extracts in mainland China. In fact, compound granule formulas that have been decocted together are presently uncommon on the Chinese domestic market. The situation is different in Taiwan and Japan, where granule formulas are generally decocted together, and whole formulas (rather than single herb extracts) form the bulk of most prescriptions. In this prescription style, whole formulas are often added as a single principle, much as one would add a single medicinal to modify a base prescription.

The prevalence of combining whole formulas together in Taiwan and Japan may be related to the fact that granule technology initially arose for creating Japanese Kampo medicines. In Japanese Kampo, whole formulas are used frequently and single medicinal extracts are rarely used. Japanese Kampo uses a smaller range of formulas than Chinese medicine, and most Kampo formulas are prescribed without modifications. Kampo formulas are frequently combined together but the addition of single medicinals or the construction of new formulas from single medicinals is uncommon.

The technology to make granules initially spread from Japan to Taiwan, where it rapidly adapted to the Chinese medical prescription style prevalent in Taiwan. Many new formulas were added to the repertoire of prepared products, and single herb extracts were added to allow for formula modifications. Taiwanese doctors have many ready–made compound formulas on the shelf to choose from, so a new prescription style based on combining whole formulas (often with single herb additions) developed there.

These variations in product availability and prescription styles have fueled different approaches in different regions. Regions that decoct formulas together tend to favor the use of compound formulas, and many practitioners in Taiwan and Japan believe that whole formulas cooked together are more effective than formulas built entirely from single extracts. Whole formulas are thought to have clear direction and succinct principles, with an eloquent balance of ingredients and an enduring historical track record. In fact, Japanese granule manufacturers must apply for arduous "new drug" applications if any aspect of a classical formula is changed, such as variation in the dose ranges of constituent medicinals.

By contrast, in mainland China the prevailing view is that combining multiple whole formulas instead of building a prescription based on single herbs causes one to include unnecessary medicinals, making the formula lose its clarity and direction. In addition, the "formula compounding" method has never been extensively evaluated clinically on the mainland because the whole formula granule products are rarely available there (the domestic market is dominated by raw herbs and single–herb granule extracts).

These diametrically opposed viewpoints have caused prescription styles to develop different regional characteristics. It is impossible to say that one approach is more effective than the other because both the mainland prescription style and the Taiwanese prescription style are routinely used in millions of patient visits.

It is not uncommon to find doctors in mainland China that do not understand the granule prescription trends in Taiwan, and many doctors in Taiwan are not aware of the new granule industry in mainland China. Since most Westerners are trained by teachers from mainland China, we often have relatively little exposure to the approach of formula combining. Thus, many practitioners have no knowledge of or experience with this method of practice.

Combining Formulas and Using Base Formulas

Using formulas as building blocks speeds the time required for dispensing, since fewer bottles need to be pulled from the shelves and fewer products need to be weighed. For example, if the pharmacy has only single herbs and Shi Quan Da Bu Tang (Ten Complete Major Supplementation Decoction) needs to be filled, 10 individual herbs must be pulled. If the whole Shi Quan Da Bu Tang formula is available, only one items needs to be weighed.

Continuing with this example, even if the whole Shi Quan Da Bu Tang formula is not stocked, it can be built from Ba Zhen Tang plus Huang Qi (astragalus) and Rou Gui (cinnamon bark). If Ba Zhen Tang is not available, it can be elaborated by combining Si Jun Zi Tang (Four Gentlemen Decoction) and Si Wu Tang (Four Agents Decoction). In this way, fewer items need to be pulled off the shelf, and one has the advantage that the ingredients have been cooked together to preserve any positive chemical interactions that may result from complete–formula–decocting.

Many of the formulas in early classical texts of Chinese medicine contained relatively few ingredients but revealed very clear principles. In particular, the eloquent ingredient combinations in Zhang Zhong–Jing's formulas from the Shang Han Lun (On Cold Damage) and the Jin Gui Yao Lue (Essential Prescriptions of the Golden Coffer) were the first records of many famous herbal combinations. These essential combinations have been elaborated to form other famous formulas for centuries, and they represent a critical aspect of the empirical evidence base of Chinese medicine. In fact, it could even be said that the herbal pairings and formulas from the Shang Han Lun and Jin Gui Yao Lue have represented one of the key areas of consensus between the medical traditions of China, Japan, and Korea up to the present day.

In many instances, the actions created by many of the basic herbal pairings in classical formulas have actually defined our modern understanding of single–herb actions and indications. For example, we now study that Chai Hu (Bupleuri Radix) resolves lesser yang, courses the liver, and raises yang, but these actions were largely developed from its employment in formulas such as Xiao Chai Hu Tang (Minor Bupleurum Decoction), Si Ni San (Counterflow Cold Powder), Chai Hu Shu Gan San (Bupleurum Liver–Coursing Powder), and Bu Zhong Yi Qi Tang (Center–Supplementing Qi–Boosting Decoction).

The small, concise formulas from early texts such as the Shang Han Lun strongly influence modern formula combining, because many of these classical formulas have a very clear therapeutic direction. In the context of the Shang Han Lun, it is not uncommon to see formulas that treat relatively severe patterns, such as the patterns associated with Si Ni Tang (Counterflow Cold Decoction) or Bai Hu Tang (White Tiger Decoction). Such formulas are rarely used on their own in the modern day, but the combinations of medicinals that they contain illustrate crucial elements of Chinese medical theory and offer great clinical efficacy.

Many of the strong classical formulas that have clear principles but are rarely indicated on their own can be incorporated into compound formulas. Illustrative examples include formulas such as Bai Hu Tang (White Tiger Decoction), Er Chen Tang (Two Matured Ingredients Decoction), Si Ni Tang (Counterflow Cold Decoction), and Huang Lian Jie Du Tang (Coptis Toxin–Resolving Decoction). These formulas are rarely used alone in an unmodified form, yet each offers a perfect unit of medicinal combinations that is succinct, focused in principle, and highly effective.

Bai Hu Tang (White Tiger Decoction)

Shi Gao (Gypsum Fibrosum)

Zhi Mu (Anemarrhenae Rhizoma)

Zhi Gan Cao (Glycyrrhizae Radix Praeparata)

Geng Mi (Oryzae Semen)

As a compound formula, Bai Hu Tang clears heat and eliminates vexation, engenders liquid and relieves thirst. It is used to treat yang brightness (*yang ming*) qi–aspect exuberant heat (also known as *yang ming* channel disease or qi–aspect heat). This presents with vigorous heat effusion, red face, vexation and thirst with taking of fluids, sweating and aversion to heat, and a flooding, large, forceful pulse.

Bai Hu Tang treats internal heat spreading throughout the whole body, with heat in both the interior and the exterior. Shi Gao is the sovereign medicinal because its great cold clears *yang ming* (qi–aspect) heat. It clears heat and eliminates vexation without damaging liquid. Zhi Mu, the minister, helps Shi Gao to clear repletion heat from the lung and stomach, and also enriches yin to engender liquid. These two medicinals have a relationship of mutual need, and their combination increases their heat–clearing and liquid–engendering power. Zhi Gan Cao and Geng Mi boost the stomach and protect liquid while preventing the cold nature of the sovereign and minister from damaging the center burner. Thus, they are both assistants and couriers.

When we look at the construction of this formula, it is obvious that the central principle lies in the combination of Shi Gao and Zhi Mu. Shi Gao and Zhi Mu complement each other with their ability to clear heat and boost liquid. These two items are powerfully cold and can be used to clear heat to treat many different disorders when they are combined with the appropriate medicinals. In the compound formula Bai Hu Tang, their cold nature is moderated by Zhi Gan Cao and Geng Mi. Thus, Bai Hu Tang is a very concise and useful formula that is perfect to use in combination with other formulas.

Bai Hu Tang is a useful formula to consider adding for cases that need a strong heat–clearing action. For example, it is common to see Bai Hu Tang with the addition of Gui Zhi (Cinnamomi Ramulus) to treat hot impediment (bi) conditions that affect the joints. Modern applications if this theory can be seen in conditions such as rheumatoid arthritis, which often manifests as a hot impediment pattern according to traditional theory.

When using Bai Hu Tang in granule form, it can also be used in small doses to increase the strength of formulas that clear lung heat. While its original indications on its own were based on treating strong heat disease, Bai Hu Tang can be used in lower doses to treat heat disease of lesser intensity. Applications include conditions such as the common cold in patients with high fever, thirst, and other symptoms of lung heat.

Similarly, Bai Hu Tang can be used to treat conditions of heat in the stomach channel. By adding Niu Xi (Achyranthis Bidentatae Radix), Sheng Di Huang (Rehmanniae Radix), and Mai Men Dong (Ophiopogonis Radix), one can essentially create the principle of the formula Yu Nu Jian (Jade Lady Brew), which is an important formula for stomach heat with yin vacuity. Bai Hu Tang can also be used with medicinals such as Huang Lian to enhance the ability of Huang Lian to clear heat in the stomach channel.

Classical modifications of Bai Hu Tang include Bai Hu Jia Ren Shen Tang (White Tiger Decoction Plus Ginseng) and Bai Hu Jia Cang Zhu Tang (White Tiger Decoction Plus Atractylodes). Both of these formulas are perfect units for a modular approach, because each formula contains potent medicinals that are combined with a clear focus and direction.

Bai Hu Jia Ren Shen Tang is a modification of the main formula that also appeared in the original Shang Han Lun. It is the same formula with the addition of Ren Shen (Ginseng Radix). This formula clears heat, boosts qi, and engenders liquid. It is indicated for basically the same presentation as the main formula, with one key difference– in this formula, while there is profuse sweating, the pulse is large but forceless because qi and liquid have been damaged. This formula may also be used for summerheat disease with damage to both qi and liquid, manifesting in sweating of the upper back, slight aversion to wind and cold, generalized heat effusion, and thirst. In wider applications, Bai Hu Jia Ren Shen Tang can be used for any of the above situations for which Bai Hu Tang is indicated, as long as there is significant qi vacuity.

If Cang Zhu (Atractylodis Rhizoma) is added, the formula clears heat and dispels dampness. It is indicated for damp–warmth disease, with generalized heat effusion, glomus in the chest, profuse sweating, and a red tongue with white greasy fur. There may also be wind–damp impediment (bì), great generalized heat effusion, and swelling and pain of the joints. This is a suitable base formula for many joint diseases that are characterized by heat and dampness.

Si Ni Tang (Counterflow Cold Decoction)

>Fu Zi (Aconiti Radix Lateralis Praeparata)
>
>Gan Jiang (Zingiberis Rhizoma)
>
>Zhi Gan Cao (Glycyrrhizae Radix Praeparata)

This simple formula is a textbook formula for warming yang. Originally indicated for shao yin disease with severe cold signs due to insufficiency of yang, this formula combines one of the most important herbal pairs for warming the interior: Gan Jiang and Fu Zi. These two hot medicinals complement each other, as the heat of Gan Jiang is said to be staying in nature while the heat of Fu Zi is mobile in nature. Gan Jiang also reduces Fu Zi's toxicity, and Zhi Gan Cao further moderates their extreme nature to harmonize the formula.

Properly combined with other medicinals and formulas, Si Ni Tang is widely applicable for conditions with yang vacuity and cold exuberance. Fu Zi used to treat all patterns of yang vacuity affecting the spleen, heart, and kidney. Granule preparations of Fu Zi are particularly useful because manufacturers utilize prolonged cooking and testing regimes to minimize its toxicity.

Si Ni Tang can be used with formulas like Si Jun Zi Tang (Four Gentlemen Decoction) to create the principle of Fu Zi Li Zhong Wan (Aconite Center–Rectifying Pill), an extremely effective formula for spleen yang vacuity.

Si Ni Tang can also be used in low doses in conjunction with formulas such as Ba Zhen Tang (Eight–Gem Decoction) for cases of qi, blood, and yang vacuity. Si Ni Tang can also be used in small quantities to enhance the treatment of yang vacuity water swelling. For cases of cold impediment, Si Ni Tang can be used as an addition to other base formulas to warm the channels and relieve pain. It can even be used in small but increasing doses to gradually transform a yin–supplementing formula such as Zuo Gui Wan (Left–Restoring Pill) into a yang–supplementing formula.

Er Chen Tang (Two Matured Ingredients Decoction)

> Ban Xia (Pinelliae Rhizoma)
>
> Chen Pi (Citri Reticulatae Pericarpium) or Ju Hong (Citri Reticulatae Pericarpium Rubrum)
>
> Fu Ling (Poria)
>
> Zhi Gan Cao (Glycyrrhizae Radix Praeparata)

Er Chen Tang is a representative base formula for patterns of dampness and phlegm. Er Chen Tang has a very clear direction and utilizes an eloquent combination of medicinals. It is thus one of the most fundamental formulas in a modular approach to formula combining, and it is very versatile when modified appropriately.

Er Chen Tang dries dampness and transforms phlegm while rectifying qi and harmonizing the center. The formula is based on the combination of Ban Xia and Chen Pi (or Ju Hong). Ban Xia is acrid, warm, and dry; it dries dampness and transforms phlegm while also harmonizing the stomach and downbearing counterflow. Chen Pi rectifies qi and moves stagnation while also drying dampness and transforming phlegm. When combined together, they are not only complementary in the sense that they increase the strength of drying dampness and transforming phlegm, but they also draw upon the principle of "[to] treat phlegm, first rectify qi, [when] qi is normalized, phlegm disperses." This combination is also the origin of the formula name, because the superior products are aged, which gives them the advantage of not being excessively dry.

Fu Ling assists by fortifying the spleen and percolating dampness, which assists the transformation of phlegm. Fortifying the spleen helps treat the origin of the dampness.

When combined with Chen Pi, the qi stagnation caused by phlegm is treated as well as the origin of the phlegm.

The addition of Sheng Jiang helps control the toxicity of Ban Xia, while also enhancing its ability to transform phlegm, harmonize the stomach, and relieve vomiting. In the original formula, a small amount of Wu Mei was used to constrain the lung qi to provide contraction within the dispersing effect and prevent damage to right from the dry, dispersing medicinals. Gan Cao fortifies the spleen and harmonizes the center, while also harmonizing the other medicinals. The overall formula is tightly constructed, and treats both root and branch, using both dispersing and constraining approaches. It dries dampness and rectifies qi to treat phlegm that is already formed, and it fortifies the spleen to treat the origin of the phlegm.

Er Chen Tang is particularly suitable to treat cases where the spleen is encumbered by dampness. Since spleen vacuity is often an underlying pathomechanism in the formation of dampness, Er Chen Tang is often combined with spleen–supplementing medicinals such as Bai Zhu (Atractylodis Macrocephalae Rhizoma) and Ren Shen (Ginseng Radix).

Er Chen Tang can also be used for vomiting in pregnancy (morning sickness). The simple addition of Zhu Ru (Bambusae Caulis in Taenia) to Er Chen Tang creates an unnamed formula from Sun Si Miao's Qian Jin Fang ("Thousand Gold Formulary") that is one of Chinese medicine's earliest formulas for vomiting in pregnancy. Further adding Huo Xiang Geng (Pogostemi Caulis), Huang Qin (Scutellariae Radix), Sang Ji Sheng (Taxilli Herba), and Xu Duan (Dipsaci Radix) to this creates a useful modern empirical formula found in major Chinese gynecology textbooks for vomiting in pregnancy.

Alternatively, Er Chen Tang can be used in combination with Si Jun Zi Tang (Four Gentlemen Decoction) to create the principle of Liu Jun Zi Tang (Six Gentlemen Decoction), which simultaneously supplements the spleen and dries dampness. Cases with more severe damp encumbrance affecting the middle burner can treated by adding Mu Xiang (Aucklandiae Radix) and Sha Ren (Amomi Fructus), creating the principle of the formula Xiang Sha Liu Jun Zi Tang (Costusroot and Amomum Six Gentlemen Decoction). These other compound formulas are available on their own, but building them from combining base formulas provides additional versatility because the dosage of the different principles (drying dampness vs. supplementing the spleen) can be adjusted based on need.

In cases where damp encumbrance is more severe than qi vacuity, medicinals such as Cang Zhu (Atractylodis Rhizoma) and Hou Po (Magnoliae Officinalis Cortex) may be added to Er Chen Tang. This brings the principle closer to the formula Ping Wei San (Stomach–Calming Powder), which treats damp obstruction of the spleen and stomach.

Er Chen Tang can also be used along with spleen–fortifying medicinals such as Bai Bian Dou (Lablab Semen Album), Bai Zhu (Atractylodis Macrocephalae Rhizoma) and Yi Yi Ren (Coicis Semen) to treat cases where spleen vacuity is present but damp obstruction is prominent. With the proper modifications, Er Chen Tang can also be used to treat conditions such as cold damp patterns of vaginal discharge as well as conditions with cold phlegm in the upper burner.

Many traditional formulas are conceptually derived from Er Chen Tang. For example, the formula Dao Tan Tang (Phlegm–Abducting Decoction) is basically Er Chen Tang plus Zhi Shi (Aurantii Fructus Immaturus) and Tian Nan Xing (Arisaematis Rhizoma), which powerfully strengthen its ability to transform phlegm. Similarly, the formula Di Tan Tang (Phlegm–Flushing Decoction) can be built from Er Chen Tang. Di Tan Tang treats wind–stroke with phlegm confounding the orifices of the heart, and basically consists of Dao Tan Tang plus Zhu Ru (Bambusae Caulis in Taenia), Shi Chang Pu (Acori Tatarinowii Rhizoma), and Ren Shen (Ginseng Radix).

Several other commonly used formulas can be easily elaborated from Er Chen Tang. Using a few base formulas to create related formulas is particularly advantageous to practitioners that have constraints on space or capital, because many formulas can be created from a small number of base formulas. In addition to the formulas mentioned above, Er Chen Tang can also be used to create formulas such as Wen Dan Tang (Gallbladder–Warming Decoction), Qing Qi Hua Tan Wan (Qi–Clearing Phlegm–Transforming Pill), and Ban Xia Bai Zhu Tian Ma Tang (Pinellia, White Atractylodes, and Gastrodia Decoction).

Wen Dan Tang (Gallbladder–Warming Decoction) is a commonly–used formula to treat the pattern of depressed gallbladder with harassing phlegm. This pattern manifests in symptoms such as susceptibility to fright, dizziness, palpitations, insomnia, frequent unusual dreams, nausea, vomiting, and epilepsy. Wen Dan Tang is created by adding Zhu Ru (Bambusae Caulis in Taenia) and Zhi Shi (Aurantii Fructus Immaturus) to Er Chen Tang. For patients with concurrent heat symptoms, Huang Lian (Coptidis Rhizoma) can be added to this to make the formula Huang Lian Wen Dan Tang (Coptis Gallbladder–Warming Decoction).

For cases of phlegm–heat cough, the formula Qing Qi Hua Tan Wan (Qi–Clearing Phlegm–Transforming Pill) can be created from Er Chen Tang. To do this, simply add Zhi Shi (Aurantii Fructus Immaturus), Gua Lou (Trichosanthis Fructus), Dan Xing (Arisaema cum Bile), and Huang Qin (Scutellariae Radix) to Er Chen Tang. These additions help the formula target phlegm–heat in the upper burner.

To treat wind–phlegm harassing the upper burner, Er Chen Tang can be modified to form the formula Ban Xia Bai Zhu Tian Ma Tang (Pinellia, White Atractylodes, and Gastrodia Decoction). This formula is an important formula for wind–phlegm patterns of headache and dizziness. It can be created by adding Bai Zhu (Atractylodis Macrocephalae Rhizoma) and Tian Ma (Gastrodiae Rhizoma) to Er Chen Tang.

The core ingredients of Er Chen Tang can be found in even more complex formulas, such as Ding Xian Wan (Fit–Settling Pill), a major formula for epilepsy. Bao He Wan (Harmony–Preserving Pill), a key formula for food stagnation, can also be elaborated from Er Chen Tang. In fact, even formulas such as Huo Xiang Zheng Qi San (Patchouli Qi–Righting Powder) can be created from a base of Er Chen Tang.

Huang Lian Jie Du Tang (Coptis Toxin–Resolving Decoction)

Huang Lian (Coptidis Rhizoma)

Huang Qin (Scutellariae Radix)

Huang Bai (Phellodendri Cortex)

Zhi Zi (Gardeniae Fructus)

Huang Lian Jie Du Tang has been an important formula in Chinese medicine since ancient times. It first appeared in the text Zhou Hou Bei Ji Fang (Emergency Standby Remedies) around the start of the 4th century AD. However, the name did not exist until it appeared in the text Wai Tai Mi Yao (Essential Secrets from Outside the Metropolis), written in 752 CE. In the modern day, Huang Lian Jie Du Tang remains one of the most important formulas for dysentery, jaundice, and various skin diseases due to damp–heat. It is also commonly used in biomedical applications for disease such as septicemia.

Huang Lian Jie Du Tang is indicated for patterns of fire toxin in all three burners. There may be great heat effusion, vexation, and agitation, as well as dry mouth and throat, disordered speech, and insomnia. Other possibilities include warm disease with vomiting of blood or nosebleed, as well as severe heat with macular eruptions, generalized heat effusion with diarrhea or dysentery, or damp–heat jaundice. In external medicine, it is used for welling–abscesses, sores, and clove sore toxin (also known as deep–rooted boils), accompanied by yellowish–red urine, a red tongue with yellow fur, and a rapid, forceful pulse.

As a full–strength decoction on its own, Huang Lian Jie Du Tang is rarely needed in modern, first–world countries. However, it is a very simple and versatile formula, and it can be used for a variety of applications in combination with other formulas. For example, it is often used to treat skin diseases due to heat toxin in combination with a formula such as Wu Wei Xiao Du Yin (Five–Ingredient Toxin–Dispersing Beverage).

Small quantities of Huang Lian Jie Du Tang can be used to modify other formulas to enhance their ability to treat damp–heat. In Taiwan, it is common to use Huang Lian Jie Du Tang in small doses in conjunction with other formulas. In fact, one can even see it used as a paradoxical assistant in warm fomulas (a paradoxical assistant is an agent used to counter the extreme nature of the primary medicinals in a formula).

For example, sometimes Taiwanese doctors use minute doses of Huang Lian Jie Du Tang with large doses of You Gui Wan (Right–Restoring Pill) when treating kidney yang vacuity. This is very counterintuitive to most practitioners, because these two formulas are completely opposite to each other in nature. Huang Lian Jie Du Tang is bitter and cold; it is used to treat damp–heat and is contraindicated in yang vacuity. By contrast, You Gui Wan is sweet and warm. It would seem that the two formulas should never be combined.

This example illustrates a key feature of formula combining. When formulas are combined, dosage is of critical importance. When supplementing yang in the hot tropical summertime of Taiwan, practitioners sometimes fear generating heat from the sweet, warm medicinals that are used to supplement yang. In raw herb prescriptions, it is common to add a single medicinal such as Huang Bai (Phellodendri Cortex) to counter this tendency. In Taiwan, some practitioners are of the opinion that adding a compound formula such as Huang Lian Jie Du Tang provides better control of any potential side effects of heat than a single medicinal addition such as Huang Bai. Consequently, one can see prescriptions that contain 5.7g of You Gui Wan and 0.3g of Huang Lian Jie

Du Tang per dose. To the untrained observer, this would appear to be a chaotic mix of opposing principles, but with proper attention to dosage this approach actually follows clear principles of Chinese medicine.

Si Ni San (Counterflow Cold Powder)

Chai Hu (Bupleuri Radix)

Zhi Shi (Aurantii Fructus Immaturus)

Bai Shao (Paeoniae Radix Alba)

Zhi Gan Cao (Glycyrrhizae Radix Praeparata)

Si Ni San was originally created to treat cold extremities due to depression of yang qi, but later generations expanded its use to treat disharmony of the liver and spleen. As such, Si Ni San is one of the most important base formulas for coursing the liver and supplementing the spleen. Si Ni San is a simple formula because it contains few ingredients, but it is profound because it contains a very eloquent combination of medicinals.

Si Ni San was one of the first formulas to combine several of the most prominent medicinal pairs in the history of Chinese medicine. Combinations of particular importance include Chai Hu with Bai Shao, Bai Shao with Zhi Gan Cao, and Chai Hu with Zhi Shi.

Wood likes orderly reaching and is averse to depression. When liver qi is depressed, it is treated with acrid, dispersing medicinals such as Chai Hu, which has an upward, floating nature. The acridity of Chai Hu accounts for its strength in coursing the liver qi, but it tends to be dry and prone to damaging yin. To counteract this tendency, it is often combined with Bai Shao, which is said to emolliate (soften) the liver. Bai Shao has a blood–nourishing effect and a sour taste that is used to check the dry, out–thrusting tendency of Chai Hu. Thus, these two medicinals are often combined, and they are routinely used together in common formulas such as Chai Hu Shu Gan San (Bupleurum Liver–Coursing Powder) and Xiao Yao San (Free Wanderer Powder).

In addition, the upbearing nature of Chai Hu is paired with the down-bearing medicinal Zhi Shi in the formula Si Ni San. Zhi Shi is a qi–moving medicinal that has a downward direction of movement, while Chai Hu is a qi–moving medicinal with an upward direction of movement. The combination of one upbearing with one downbearing medicinal in the formula Si Ni San is important, because these two medicinals use their complementary opposition to increase the overall movement of qi while checking each other's extreme tendencies. Just as Chai Hu and Bai Shao combine acridity with sourness (and their corresponding dispersing and constraining natures), Chai Hu and Zhi Shi reinforce each other in the goal of moving qi.

The combination of Bai Shao with Zhi Gan Cao is also important in Si Ni San. In fact, the combination of these two medicinals constitutes a formula known as Shao Yao Gan Cao Tang (Peony and Licorice Decoction), which is a major formula for calf spasms. Bai Shao and Zhi Gan Cao are used together to treat spasmodic, cramping pain throughout the body, and they are particularly effective for cramping pain in the abdomen as well.

Si Ni San is a very useful starting point for many conditions that are due to a disharmony of wood and earth. For wood–earth disharmony manifesting in painful diarrhea, Si Ni San can be combined with the compound formula Tong Xie Yao Fang (Pain and Diarrhea Formula). In modern Chinese medicine, this combination is very common for treating patients with irritable bowel syndrome (IBS) when the case manifests with cramping pain and diarrhea due to a wood–earth disharmony.

Tong Xie Yao Fang is itself a formula for harmonizing wood and earth. Rather than using Chai Hu to course the liver, it uses the acrid nature of Fang Feng (Saposhnikoviae Radix), which is less drying. Chinese formula texts also often emphasize that Fang Feng is aromatic, which helps to guide the formula to the spleen. Tong Xie Yao Fang also contains Chen Pi (Citri Reticulatae Pericarpium) and Bai Zhu (Atractylodis Macrocephalae Rhizoma), which makes it slightly more suitable for treating spleen vacuity complicated by dampness. Tong Xie Yao Fang and Si Ni San share the presence of Bai Shao. The two formulas can be combined together, or one can simply add Chen Pi (Citri Reticulatae Pericarpium), Fang Feng (Saposhnikoviae Radix), and Bai Zhu (Atractylodis Macrocephalae Rhizoma) to Si Ni San.

To take Si Ni San in a different direction, the liver–coursing effect of Si Ni San can be strengthened by adding acrid medicinals such as Xiang Fu (Cyperi Rhizoma) and Chuan Xiong (Chuanxiong Rhizoma). These medicinals appear together in the formula Chai Hu Shu Gan San (Bupleurum Liver–Coursing Powder), which is itself an eloquent formula for treating binding depression of liver qi.

The formula Chai Hu Shu Gan San can also be expanded by adding medicinals such as Hong Hua (Carthami Flos) and Tao Ren (Persicae Semen) to combine the principles of coursing liver qi and quickening the blood. These principles are often combined because stagnation of qi tends to lead to stagnation of blood, and quickening the blood is best accomplished by simultaneously moving qi. Such modifications are particularly common in the field of gynecology, because conditions such as menstrual pain are often associated with liver depression and blood stasis.

Continuing in the direction of blood–quickening, the formula Xue Fu Zhu Yu Tang (Expelling Stasis in the House of Blood Decoction) and its own derivative formulas can be created from a base of either Si Ni San or Chai Hu Shu Gan San. This opens up an entire category of qi– and blood–moving formulas. For example, medicinals such as Pu Huang (Typhae Pollen), Wu Ling Zhi (Trogopteri Faeces), and Yan Hu Suo (Corydalis Rhizoma) can be added to relieve pain due to blood stasis, a principle also found in the formula Ge Xia Zhu Yu Tang (Infradiaphragmatic Stasis–Expelling Decoction).

In Chai Hu Shu Gan San, the liver–coursing effect of Si Ni San is accentuated. By contrast, if the spleen–fortifying aspect of Si Ni San is accentuated by the addition of medicinals such as Bai Zhu (Atractylodis Macrocephalae Rhizoma) and Fu Ling (Poria), the formula moves in the direction of Xiao Yao San (Free Wanderer Powder). Xiao Yao San is a formula that strikes a harmonious balance between coursing wood and gently supplementing earth and blood.

Xiao Yao San itself is an important base formula in modular approaches to formula combining. Like Si Ni San, Xiao Yao San can be used in combination with other formulas or can be easily elaborated to form related classical formulas or their derivatives.

Xiao Yao San (Free Wanderer Powder)

Chai Hu (Bupleuri Radix)

Bai Shao (Paeoniae Radix Alba)

Dang Gui (Angelicae Sinensis Radix)

Bai Zhu (Atractylodis Macrocephalae Rhizoma)

Fu Ling (Poria)

Sheng Jiang (Zingiberis Rhizoma Recens) [roasted]

Bo He (Menthae Herba)

Gan Cao (Glycyrrhizae Radix)

Xiao Yao San is one of the most commonly prescribed formulas in Chinese medicine. According to research conducted by Dr. Chang Hsien–Cheh of China Medical University on Taiwan's National Health Insurance data, doctors in Taiwan prescribed 14.1 metric tons of granule Xiao Yao San between the years of 2003 and 2004. One of its related formulas, Jia Wei Xiao Yao San, was prescribed in a stunning quantity of 86.3 metric tons during the same time period.

The formula Xiao Yao San strikes an even balance between coursing the liver and supplementing the spleen. The acrid, potent liver qi–coursing medicinal Chai Hu is complemented by Bo He, which has a gentle ability to course the liver qi. The dry, acrid, and dispersing nature of Chai Hu is offset by the sweet, blood–nourishing medicinals Bai Shao and Dang Gui. Fu Ling, Bai Zhu, and Gan Cao supplement the spleen to protect earth from being exploited by wood, an essential aspect of treating wood–earth disharmony.

From a base of Xiao Yao San, many additional formulas can be created. For example, the formula Jia Wei Xiao Yao San (Augmented Free Wanderer Powder, also known as Dan Zhi Xiao Yao San) is easily created by adding Mu Dan Pi (Moutan Cortex) and Zhi Zi (Gardeniae Fructus). This gives the formula a heat–clearing effect, which is useful for cases where liver depression forms heat. Like Xiao Yao San itself, the formula Jia Wei Xiao Yao San is a major formula in gynecology and has widespread applications throughout internal medicine.

With the addition of rehmannia to Xiao Yao San, the formula Hei Xiao

Yao San (Black Free Wanderer Powder) is formed. Hei Xiao Yao San can be made by adding either Sheng Di Huang (Rehmanniae Radix) or Shu Di Huang (Rehmanniae Radix Praeparata) to Xiao Yao San. This formula is used for cases with more prominent blood vacuity. If there is more heat in the blood, use Sheng Di Huang. If there is more blood vacuity, use Shu Di Huang.

In the method of formula combining commonly seen in Taiwan, compound formulas are often used as a single principle, much as one would consider the addition of a single medicinal when making a raw formula. An entire formula is added to modify the prescription, which allows for more choices than one has with single medicinals alone. For example, no single medicinal offers the simultaneous action of coursing the liver, supplementing the spleen, and nourishing the blood. However, if whole formulas are used to modify a prescription, the formula Xiao Yao San provides this entire conceptual unit.

Depending on whether the dosage is high or low, Xiao Yao San can be used as either the main prescription or as a modification. For example, Dr. Feng Ye, a prominent expert clinician in Taiwan, has been known to widely use Xiao Yao San as an addition to many base formulas for the purpose of balancing the qi dynamic between wood and earth. In cases where wood–earth disharmony is the primary problem, Dr. Feng will use 12–18 grams per day of Xiao Yao San. For cases where wood–earth disharmony is not the main pattern being treated but remains an accessory concern, Dr. Feng will use Xiao Yao San in a dosage of 1–4 grams per day, in conjunction with other formulas that treat the principle pattern. He also has extensive experience incorporating harmonizing formulas such as Xiao Chai Hu Tang (Minor Bupleurum Decoction) and Jia Wei Xiao Yao San (Augmented Free Wanderer Powder) in similar ways, depending on the constitution of the patient.

To explore another illustrative example of Dr. Feng's clinical formula combining with Xiao Yao San, consider one of his treatment strategies for constipation. Constipation can result from many pathomechanisms in Chinese medicine, all of which require different treatments. However, one presentation that is particularly common in young people, especially young women, is the pattern of mild constipation due to liver depression or a wood–earth disharmony. For such cases, Dr. Feng has successfully employed the combination of Xiao Yao San with Ma Zi Ren Wan (Cannabis Seed Pill).

In this example, Xiao Yao San is able to treat the root cause of mild liver depression, but it lacks the specific action of freeing the stool. Ma Zi Ren Wan is able to treat the symptom of constipation but it lacks the ability to treat the root pattern of liver depression. When the two formulas are combined, both symptomatic and root treatment is achieved. Over time, the symptomatic contribution of Ma Zi Ren Wan can be reduced relative to the root treatment of regulating wood and earth, allowing the Ma Zi Ren Wan to be tapered off and gradually eliminated as the core pattern resolves. Clinically, this strategy starts with a daily dose of about 12 grams of Xiao Yao San and 2–6 grams of Ma Zi Ren Wan. Over the course of a few weeks, the dose of the Ma Zi Ren Wan can be gradually reduced and the Xiao Yao San can be gradually increased, until eventually the Ma Zi Ren Wan is no longer used and the patient achieves normal bowel movements with the root formula of Xiao Yao San alone.

Gui Zhi Tang (Cinnamon Twig Decoction)

> Gui Zhi (Cinnamomi Ramulus)
>
> Bai Shao (Paeoniae Radix Alba)
>
> Da Zao (Jujubae Fructus)
>
> Sheng Jiang (Zingiberis Rhizoma Recens)
>
> Zhi Gan Cao (Glycyrrhizae Radix Praeparata)

Gui Zhi Tang is a formula from the Shang Han Lun ("On Cold Damage") that was originally indicated for greater yang wind strike patterns of cold damage. The combination of medicinals within Gui Zhi Tang is very eloquent and subtle variations in additions can take the formula in several new directions. Gui Zhi Tang is essentially a formula for balancing yin and yang, and it is one of the most balanced and profound formulas within Chinese medicine.

Gui Zhi Tang relies on the complementary opposition of Gui Zhi and Bai Shao. Gui Zhi is warm and outward moving, which Bai Shao is cool and constraining in action. The construction–defense disharmony that is treated in Gui Zhi Tang is essentially an imbalance of yin and yang, here expressed as an imbalance between construction and defense, or the interior and the exterior. The warm freeing action of Gui Zhi treats the yang aspect of the problem (defense) while the nourishing and consolidating action of Bai Shao treats the yin aspect of the problem (construction). Together, they balance the interior and exterior and harmonize yin and yang. Traditionally, this is explained through the use of a military analogy, with Bai Shao representing the "camp" or supply and Gui Zhi representing the "defense" or the troops at the perimeter.

Beyond Gui Zhi and Bai Shao, Gui Zhi Tang also contains a unit of earth–supplementing medicinals that appear together in many other Shang Han Lun formulas. These medicinals also rely on mutual opposition; the acrid, dispersing nature of Sheng Jiang prevents the sweet, rich nature of Da Zao from causing stagnation, while Zhi Gan Cao both supplements the spleen and harmonizes the formula.

Chinese formula texts state that Gui Zhi Tang is indicated for external contraction of wind–cold with exterior vacuity and disharmony of construction and defense. This pattern is characterized by headache, heat effusion, aversion to wind, and sweating, possibly accompanied by "noisy nose" (nasal congestion with audible breathing), absence of thirst, and/or dry retching.

Under normal physiologic conditions, defense qi moves outside the vessels and secures and protects the fleshy exterior. Construction–yin stays inside and provides nourishment to defense yang, and construction and defense are in harmony.

In the pathologic state addressed by Gui Zhi Tang, vacuity of defense qi causes the interstices to be loose. Defense yang cannot secure and protect the fleshy exterior, so there is aversion to cold. Construction–yin cannot stay in the inner body and discharges outward, causing sweating. The combination of Gui Zhi (Cinnamomi Ramulus) and Bai Shao (Paeoniae Radix Alba) both dissipates and contracts. This allows evil to be dispelled without damaging right while simultaneously nourishing yin without lodging evil.

Gui Zhi Tang is said to "transform qi and regulate yin and yang," and it is used for miscellaneous diseases in internal medicine that are ascribed to disharmony of yin and yang, construction and defense, or qi and blood. It is especially suitable for conditions following illness or childbirth, or for generalized weakness when the chief manifestations are aversion to wind and sweating.

Within the original Shang Han Lun, there are uses of Gui Zhi Tang that do not manifest with greater yang wind–strike. For example, it is mentioned for patients with periodic heat effusion and spontatneous sweating, in the absence of other visceral diseases. Here, it is taken prior to the onset of heat effusion to harmonize construction and defense.

Gui Zhi Tang is contraindicated in patients with greater yang cold damage signs. Because it is too mild in comparison with Ma Huang Tang (Ephedra Decoction), one will miss the best opportunity for dispelling evil.

Gui Zhi Tang is also contraindicated in interior damp–heat patterns. This is alluded to in the Shang Han Lun in a discussion of its adverse effects on "sick drinkers." The formula is acrid and sweet, and acrid flavors reinforce heat and sweet flavors reinforce dampness, so there is a general caution against the use of Gui Zhi Tang in the interior damp–heat conditions. The original meaning of the phrase "sick drinkers" (*jiu ke bing*) is unclear, it may refer either to a disease name (drinker's sickness, i.e., alcoholism) or to a drinker (*jiu ke*) who is sick. If it refers to the latter, it is unclear whether they are sick with greater yang wind–strike or sick from drinking. Different sources draw different conclusions about this statement.

Gui Zhi Tang is also inappropriate for patients with exuberant interior heat, as well as in greater yang disease that has been erroneously treated with purging and no exterior signs remain present.

The addition of Ge Gen (Puerariae Radix) to this formula modifies it to treat hypertonicity in the nape and back. This is a pattern of simultaneous greater yang wind strike and constrained greater yang channel qi.

The fluids are damaged and cannot moisten and nourish the channels normally.

To treat variations of wind–cold with Gui Zhi Tang, consider the following modifications:

For marked insufficiency of defense yang with prominent aversion to cold, increase the quantity of Gui Zhi and Gan Cao, or add Fu Zi (Aconiti Radix Lateralis Praeparata).

For incessant leaking sweat in cases of relatively severe defense qi vacuity, add Huang Qi (Astragali Radix) and Bai Zhu (Atractylodis Macrocephalae Rhizoma).

For profuse sweating and a thin pulse from weakness of construction, increase the dose of Bai Shao and Gan Cao.

From a base of Gui Zhi Tang, several other important formulas can be created, such as Xiao Jian Zhong Tang (Minor Center–Fortifying Decoction), Huang Qi Jian Zhong Tang (Astragalus Center–Fortifying Decoction), Ge Gen Tang (Pueraria Decoction), and Gui Zhi Jia Long Gu Mu Li Tang (Cinnamon Twig Decoction Plus Dragon Bone and Oyster Shell).

Xiao Jian Zhong Tang (Minor Center–Fortifying Decoction)

Gui Zhi (Cinnamomi Ramulus)

Bai Shao (Paeoniae Radix Alba)

Da Zao (Jujubae Fructus)

Sheng Jiang (Zingiberis Rhizoma Recens)

Zhi Gan Cao (Glycyrrhizae Radix Praeparata)

Yi Tang (Maltosum)

The profound nature of Gui Zhi Tang is readily apparent because of the dramatic change in indications achieved by subtle modifications, in this case the simple addition of Yi Tang (Maltosum). While Gui Zhi Tang is a formula for external contraction, Xiao Jian Zhong Tang is a major formula for internal medicine. Specifically, Xiao Jian Zhong Tang is a representative formula for vacuity cold patterns of abdominal pain, among other indications.

Yi Tang is a sweet medicinal that supplements the center and "relaxes tension." The action of "relaxing tension" (*huan ji*) only appears in three common items in the Chinese materia medica: Yi Tang, Bai Shao, and Gan Cao. All three of these medicinals are used together in the formula Xiao Jian Zhong Tang, which accounts for its profound ability to treat cramping pain in vacuity patterns. The warm nature of Gui Zhi allows the formula to be suitable for cold patterns, and the sweet, supplementing action of the other medicinals makes Xiao Jian Zhong Tang suitable for vacuity patterns.

For cases with more significant qi vacuity, Huang Qi (Astragali Radix) may be added to Xiao Jian Zhong Tang. This forms the formula Huang Qi Jian Zhong Tang (Astragalus Center–Fortifying Decoction), which is also an important formula for qi vacuity patterns of abdominal pain.

Ge Gen Tang (Pueraria Decoction)

> Gui Zhi (Cinnamomi Ramulus)
>
> Bai Shao (Paeoniae Radix Alba)
>
> Da Zao (Jujubae Fructus)
>
> Sheng Jiang (Zingiberis Rhizoma Recens)
>
> Zhi Gan Cao (Glycyrrhizae Radix Praeparata)
>
> Ge Gen (Puerariae Radix)
>
> Ma Huang (Ephedrae Herba)

Ge Gen Tang is a major formula for common cold. In fact, it is the most commonly used OTC herbal formula in Japan for treating common cold. Ge Gen Tang can be formed from Gui Zhi Tang by simply adding Ma Huang and Ge Gen, and it combines the principles of both Ma Huang Tang (Ephedra Decoction) and Gui Zhi Tang. It is also sometimes used in Chinese medical traumatology to treat muscular pain of the upper back and neck (Gui Zhi Tang plus Ge Gen alone can be used here as well).

Ge Gen Tang promotes sweating and resolves the exterior, engenders liquid and soothes the channels. By combining Gui Zhi with Ma Huang, its ability to enhance sweating is accentuated. This makes it applicable for repletion patterns of wind–cold. The addition of Ge Gen also makes the formula suitable for treating stiff neck and diarrhea.

Ge Gen Tang has several main applications. It is indicated for greater yang (*tai yang*) disease with "stretched stiff nape and back," absence of sweating, and aversion to wind. Stretched stiff nape and back refers to hypertonicity of the neck and back and discomfort when looking up and down, as if the neck were forcefully stretched, a condition that is considered more severe than simple stiffness and pain in the neck.

Ge Gen Tang is also used for greater yang (tai yang) and yang brightness (*yang ming*) combination disease, manifesting with diarrhea. The original text describes this as "spontaneous diarrhea," meaning that it is diarrhea that occurs without any known natural or iatrogenic cause (such as inappropriate purging). This pattern is one of simultaneous disease in the interior and exterior, with the exterior aspect being the most significant.

Gui Zhi Jia Long Gu Mu Li Tang (Cinnamon Twig Decoction Plus Dragon Bone and Oyster Shell)

Gui Zhi (Cinnamomi Ramulus)

Bai Shao (Paeoniae Radix Alba)

Da Zao (Jujubae Fructus)

Sheng Jiang (Zingiberis Rhizoma Recens)

Zhi Gan Cao (Glycyrrhizae Radix Praeparata)

Long Gu (Mastodi Ossis Fossilia)

Mu Li (Ostreae Concha)

Gui Zhi Jia Long Gu Mu Li Tang is a formula that is created by adding Long Gu (Mastodi Ossis Fossilia) and Mu Li (Ostreae Concha) to Gui Zhi Tang. This formula harmonizes yin and yang, subdues with heavy settling and secures and astringes. This formula is based on the concept of harmonizing yin and yang that underlies most of the Gui Zhi Tang derivative formulas. Gui Zhi Jia Long Gu Mu Li Tang is particularly concerned with promoting interaction of the heart (fire) and kidney (water).

If yin depletion affects yang, there will be dual vacuity of yin and yang. Kidney and heart cannot interact; in men there will be seminal emission or seminal efflux, in women there is dreaming of intercourse with ghosts. There may be hypertonicity of the lesser abdomen, cold pain of the genitals, dizziness and loss of hair, spontaneous sweating or night sweating, heart palpitations and insomnia, pale red tongue with thin white fur, and a thin weak or thin slow pulse. Gui Zhi Jia Long Gu Mu Li Tang is indicated in such conditions.

Si Wu Tang (Four Substances Decoction)

> Dang Gui (Angelicae Sinensis Radix)
>
> Bai Shao (Paeoniae Radix Alba)
>
> Shu Di Huang (Rehmanniae Radix Praeparata)
>
> Chuan Xiong (Chuanxiong Rhizoma)

Si Wu Tang is an important blood–supplementing formula in Chinese medicine, and it is particularly suitable for use in a modular approach to formula combining. Si Wu Tang is one of the most famous formulas throughout East Asian society because it is often incorporated into medicinal soups and OTC products. Within it, the rich blood–supplementing medicinals are complemented by the acrid, blood–quickening nature of Chuan Xiong, which helps to prevent stagnation when nourishing the blood.

Si Wu Tang can be combined with the formula Si Jun Zi Tang (Four Gentlemen Decoction) to simultaneously supplement qi and blood. The combination of these two formulas forms Ba Zhen Tang (Eight Gem Decoction). If one makes Ba Zhen Tang from the combination of Si Wu Tang and Si Jun Zi Tang, the relative proportions of qi–supplementing medicinals vs. blood–supplementing can be easily adjusted.

The further addition of Huang Qi (Astragali Radix) and Rou Gui (Cinnamomi Cortex) to Ba Zhen Tang creates the formula Shi Quan Da Bu Tang (Perfect Major Supplementation Decoction). This gives the formula a slightly warmer nature, and takes advantage of the ability of Rou Gui to enhance the generation of qi and blood. Here, Huang Qi strongly supplements the spleen and its combination with Dang Gui forms another formula unit, Dang Gui Bu Xue Tang (Chinese Angelica Blood–Supplementing Decoction).

If Si Wu Tang is instead combined with Hong Hua (Carthami Flos) and Tao Ren (Persicae Semen), the formula Tao Hong Si Wu Tang (Peach Kernel and Carthamus Four Substances Decoction) is formed. Tao Hong Si Wu Tang typically also involves the substitution of Chi Shao (Paeoniae Radix Rubra) in place of Bai Shao (Paeoniae Radix Alba) and Dang Gui Wei (Angelicae Sinensis Radicis Extremitas) in place of Dang Gui (Angelicae Sinensis Radix). While this substitution is often desirable, the formula is still viable without substituting these ingredients—Dang Gui Wei and Dang Gui are largely the same in terms of their chemical constituents, and Chi Shao and Bai Shao were used interchangeably for centuries (in fact, the species used as Bai Shao is sold as Chi Shao when it is wild–harvested to this day).

Adding E Jiao (Asini Corii Colla), Ai Ye (Artemisiae Argyi Folium), and Gan Cao (Glycyrrhizae Radix) to Si Wu Tang creates the formula Jiao Ai Tang (Ass Hide Glue and Mugwort Decoction). Jiao Ai Tang was one of the first formulas in the field of Chinese medical gynecology, preceding Si Wu Tang itself. It treats prolonged menstruation, flooding and spotting, and incessant bleeding due to spontaneous abortion or childbirth. Jiao Ai Tang is also used for threatened miscarriage with bleeding during pregnancy, with soreness and pain of the lower abdomen. Jiao Ai Tang nourishes the blood and stanches bleeding, and also regulates menstruation and quiets the fetus. It is indicated for patterns of vacuity detriment of the thoroughfare (*chong*) and controlling (*ren*) vessels, and patterns of blood vacuity with cold.

If Ren Shen (Ginseng Radix) and Huang Qi (Astragali Radix) are added to Si Wu Tang, the formula Sheng Yu Tang (Sagacious Cure Decoction) is formed. This formula supplements qi and blood and contains the blood. It is used for qi and blood vacuity patterns where qi fails to control the blood, manifesting in early menstruation with profuse bleeding of pale blood.

Xiao Cheng Qi Tang (Minor Qi–Coordinating Decoction)

Da Huang (Rhei Radix et Rhizoma)

Zhi Shi (Aurantii Fructus Immaturus)

Hou Po (Magnoliae Officinalis Cortex)

Xiao Cheng Qi Tang is an important base formula for constipation. It is relatively strong on its own at full–strength doses, but it is very versatile for formula combining when it is used in small quantities. In fact, Xiao Cheng Qi Tang is itself found in other formulas, such as Ma Zi Ren Wan (Cannabis Seed Pill).

Xiao Cheng Qi Tang is part of one of the oldest formula families in Chinese medicine, most of which came from the chapter on yang brightness (yang ming) disease in the *Shang Han Lun (On Cold Damage)*. For repletion cases of heat constipation manifesting with dryness, hardness, glomus, and fullness, Mang Xiao (Natrii Sulfas) can be added to Xiao Cheng Qi Tang to form its parent formula, Da Cheng Qi Tang (Major Qi–Coordinating Decoction).

In cases where there is depletion of yin–humor, the formula Zeng Ye Tang (Humor–Increasing Decoction) can be combined with Xiao Cheng Qi Tang to form a formula that is somewhat similar to Zeng Ye Cheng Qi Tang (Humor–Increasing Qi–Coordinating Decoction). Xiao Cheng Qi Tang can also be added to formulas such as Bao He Wan (Harmony–Preserving Pill) for severe food stagnation with constipation.

For more mild cases of constipation, the formula Xiao Cheng Qi Tang can be modified by adding Huo Ma Ren (Cannabis Semen), Bai Shao (Paeoniae Radix Alba), Xing Ren (Armeniacae Semen), and Feng Mi (Mel). This forms the formula Ma Zi Ren Wan (Cannabis Seed Pill), which is itself an excellent building block for treating constipation within the formula combining approach.

Xiao Chai Hu Tang (Minor Bupleurum Decoction)

Chai Hu (Bupleuri Radix)

Huang Qin (Scutellariae Radix)

Ren Shen (Ginseng Radix)

Zhi Gan Cao (Glycyrrhizae Radix Praeparata)

Ban Xia (Pinelliae Rhizoma)

Sheng Jiang (Zingiberis Rhizoma Recens)

Da Zao (Jujubae Fructus)

Xiao Chai Hu Tang is an excellent base formula to build from because it harmonizes wood and earth and also regulates upbearing and downbearing. Its core medicinal combination of Huang Qin and Chai Hu allows it to harmonize lesser yang, and its supporting medicinals are very gracefully combined.

When wood is depressed, earth will be influenced, causing the spleen and stomach to lose their normal upbearing and downbearing. Here, Ban Xia deals with depressed fluids from poor movement and transformation. By transforming pathological fluids, usable fluids may be diffused and normal downbearing may be restored. In complementary opposition, Ren Shen engenders liquid and promotes the spleen's normal upbearing.

By regulating wood and earth as well as upbearing and downbearing, Xiao Chai Hu Tang can be used as a starting point for a stunning variety of conditions. It is a model of balanced formula construction, displaying a nice balance between supplementing and dispersing, dry and moist medicinals, and warm and cold medicinals. The importance of Xiao Chai Hu Tang cannot be underestimated, and it has proven to be one of the most important and versatile formulas in Chinese medicine. It is also one of the most commonly prescribed formulas in modern Japanese Kampo, where it is used for hepatitis and many other disorders.

Long Dan Xie Gan Tang (Gentian Liver–Draining Decoction)

Long Dan Cao (Gentianae Radix)

Huang Qin (Scutellariae Radix)

Zhi Zi (Gardeniae Fructus)

Chai Hu (Bupleuri Radix)

Dang Gui (Angelicae Sinensis Radix)

Sheng Di Huang (Rehmanniae Radix)

Che Qian Zi (Plantaginis Semen)

Ze Xie (Alismatis Rhizoma)

Mu Tong (Akebiae Trifoliatae Caulis)

Gan Cao (Glycyrrhizae Radix)

Long Dan Xie Gan Tang is a very important formula. It has two major applications: upward flaming of liver–gallbladder repletion fire, and patterns of liver channel damp–heat pouring downward.

Upward flaming of liver–gallbladder repletion fire may present with headache and red eyes, rib–side pain, bitter taste in the mouth, deafness, swelling of the ear, a red tongue with yellow fur, and a wiry, rapid, and forceful pulse. Liver channel damp–heat pouring downward manifests in swelling of the genitals, itching of the genitals, wilting of the sinews, sweating of the genitals, turbid strangury, or yellow foul–smelling vaginal discharge. The tongue is red with yellow greasy fur, and the pulse is wiry, rapid, and forceful.

This formula has several special features. It combines the use of clearing and draining with percolating and disinhibiting, and drains liver fire above while disinhibiting damp–heat below. It has a balance of opposing principles: Within its draining, it includes supplementing, and although it disinhibits, it also enriches. Within its downbearing, there is upbearing, and it dispels evil without damaging right. Nonetheless, it is still considered a bitter, cold formula that easily damages the spleen and stomach.

Within the formula, Long Dan Cao clears repletion fire from the liver and gallbladder, and also treats damp–heat in the liver and gallbladder. Huang Qin and Zhi Zi drain fire and dry dampness, assisting Long Dan Cao in its ability to drain liver fire, dry dampness, and clear heat. Ze Xie, Mu Tong, and Che Qian Zi clear heat and disinhibit dampness, causing damp–heat to move downward to be eliminated via the waterways. Sheng Di Huang and Dang Gui supplement blood and yin to prevent liver heat from damaging yin and blood. This provides supplementing within drainage and prevents the bitter–drying and percolating–disinhibiting medicinals from damaging yin. Chai Hu courses the liver and clears heat; by coursing qi, it resolves depressed heat. It also conducts the medicinals into the liver and gallbladder, so it has a concurrent role as a courier. Gan Cao clears heat and harmonizes all the medicinals.

Long Dan Xie Gan Tang is a very versatile formula within the formula combining paradigm. In the context of internal medicine, repletion heat or damp–heat affecting the liver–gallbladder often calls for Long Dan Xie Gan Tang, but some conditions use different additions to modify its focus. For example, it is common to combine Cang Er Zi San (Xanthium Powder) with Long Dan Xie Gan Tang to treat deep–source nasal congestion in cases due to depressed heat in the gallbladder channel.

One interesting application of Long Dan Xie Gan Tang in formula combining can be seen from the following example. In an effort to develop effective treatments for endometriosis, practitioners at Chang Gung Memorial Hospital in Taiwan investigated the appearance of endometrial tissue obtained by a diagnostic biopsy. By using a microscope to examine the tissue, they were able to gather information that was not available to practitioners in the past. One of their findings was that the tissue was typically red and inflamed. Looking through the lens of Chinese medicine, this appeared to be a clear manifestation of heat that may not have been visible via conventional intake methods. In cases where the tissue was proliferating locally, the location of this heat could be placed on the liver channel.

This discovery spurred many doctors to experiment with the use of Long Dan Xie Gan Tang in their patients with endometriosis. For patients that lack a true damp–heat presentation, the cold nature of the base formula may be adjusted by combining it with a warm, spleen–supporting formula such as Xiang Sha Liu Jun Zi Tang (Costusroot and Amomum Six Gentlemen Decoction). Practitioners who use this novel method may use different base formulas depending on the patient's presentation, with a relatively minor quantity of Long Dan Xie Gan Tang added in. While such a strategy is the subject of debate, it is an interesting example of the Taiwanese method of formula combining.

Liu Wei Di Huang Wan (Six–Ingredient Rehmannia Pill)

Shu Di Huang (Rehmanniae Radix Praeparata)

Shan Zhu Yu (Corni Fructus)

Shan Yao (Dioscoreae Rhizoma)

Fu Ling (Poria)

Ze Xie (Alismatis Rhizoma)

Mu Dan Pi (Moutan Cortex)

Liu Wei Di Huang Wan is one of the most famous formulas for supplementing yin. It is relatively mild and harmonious because of its balance of "three supplementing" and "three draining" medicinals, and it is easily modified to form other related formulas.

One of the most commonly prescribed formulas for clearing vacuity heat is Zhi Bai Di Huang Wan (Anemarrhena, Phellodendron, and Rehmannia Pill), which is formed by adding Zhi Mu (Anemarrhenae Rhizoma) and Huang Bai (Phellodendri Cortex) to Liu Wei Di Huang Wan.

By contrast, the addition of Fu Zi (Aconiti Radix Lateralis Praeparata) and Rou Gui (Cinnamomi Cortex) or Gui Zhi (Cinnamomi Ramulus) to Liu Wei Di Huang Wan forms the yang–supplementing formula Shen Qi Wan (Kidney Qi Pill). This formula is particularly useful for treating patterns of water swelling due to kidney yang vacuity, and it can be used as a base for a wide range of yang–supplementing applications. For example, it can be further elaborated by adding Zi He Che (Hominis Placenta), Mai Men Dong (Ophiopogonis Radix), Lu Rong (Cervi Cornu Pantotrichum), and Wu Wei Zi (Schisandrae Fructus). This forms the formula He Che Ba Wei Wan (Eight–Ingredient Placenta Pill), a powerful qi–, blood–, yin– and yang–supplementing formula.

If Wu Wei Zi (Schisandrae Fructus) and Mai Men Dong (Ophiopogonis Radix) are added to Liu Wei Di Huang Wan, the formula Mai Wei Di Huang Wan (Ophiopogon and Rehmannia Pill) is formed. Alternatively, the addition of Wu Wei Zi, Ci Shi (Magnetitum), and Chai Hu (Bupleuri Radix) to Liu Wei Di Huang Wan creates the formula Er Long Zuo Ci Wan (Deafness Left–Benefiting Loadstone Pill), which is a major formula for tinnitus and deafness.

Additional possibilities for modifying Liu Wei Di Huang Wan include adding medicinals such as Ju Hua (Chrysanthemi Flos) and Gou Qi Zi (Lycii Fructus) to form Qi Ju Di Huang Wan (Lycium Berry, Chrysanthemum, and Rehmannia Pill). This formula supplements the liver and kidney and brightens the eyes. By further adding Shi Jue Ming (Haliotidis Concha), Bai Ji Li (Tribuli Fructus), Bai Shao (Paeoniae Radix Alba), and Dang Gui (Angelicae Sinensis Radix), one can make the empirical formula Ming Mu Di Huang Wan (Eye-Brightener Rehmannia Pill), which also brightens the eyes.

Small Formula Units

Beyond using major base formulas as a starting point to treat the main pattern, adding small formula units is an important aspect of the formula combining approach. Often, small, succinct formulas contain very concise and targeted combinations of medicinals that are perfect for achieving resolution of specific symptoms or secondary patterns. Below are several examples of formulas that can be easily incorporated into a modular approach.

Er Miao San (Mysterious Two Powder)

> Cang Zhu (Atractylodis Rhizoma)
>
> Huang Bai (Phellodendri Cortex)

San Miao San (Mysterious Three Powder)

> Cang Zhu (Atractylodis Rhizoma)
>
> Huang Bai (Phellodendri Cortex)
>
> Niu Xi (Achyranthis Bidentatae Radix)

Si Miao San (Mysterious Four Powder)

> Cang Zhu (Atractylodis Rhizoma)
>
> Huang Bai (Phellodendri Cortex)
>
> Niu Xi (Achyranthis Bidentatae Radix)
>
> Yi Yi Ren (Coicis Semen)

Er Miao San (Mysterious Two Powder) and its related formulas, San Miao San (Mysterious Three Powder) and Si Miao San (Mysterious Four Powder), are all extremely useful formulas for patterns of damp–heat. When combined appropriately, these formulas can be used to treat a wide variety of conditions, ranging from hot impediment patterns (especially affecting the lower body) to conditions such as damp–heat patterns of vaginal discharge.

Dang Gui Bu Xue Tang (Chinese Angelica Blood–Supplementing Decoction)

> Dang Gui (Angelicae Sinensis Radix)
>
> Huang Qi (Astragali Radix)

Dang Gui Bu Xue Tang is a small formula that uses a high dose of Huang Qi to strongly supplement qi to encourage the generation of blood. On its own, it is originally indicated for blood loss, but it can be added to many other formulas to enhance the base formula's ability to supplement qi and blood. Dang Gui Bu Xue Tang appears within other compound formulas such as Gui Pi Tang (Spleen–Returning Decoction) and Shi Quan Da Bu Tang (Major Supplementation Decoction), and it is a very useful conceptual unit for a modular approach to formula combining.

Mu Li San (Oyster Shell Powder)

> Mu Li (Ostreae Concha)
>
> Ma Huang Gen (Ephedrae Radix)
>
> Huang Qi (Astragali Radix)

Mu Li San secures the exterior and constrains sweat. It is indicated for vacuity patterns of spontaneous sweating or night sweating. Mu Li San is a representative formula for frequent spontaneous sweating that is especially severe at night and is enduring and incessant, possibly accompanied by palpitations and fright, shortness of breath, vexation and fatigue.

Sweating is differentiated based on night sweating and spontaneous sweating. Spontaneous sweating occurs outside of sleep and is not caused by movement or taxation. Night sweating (literally "thief sweating") occurs while asleep. Spontaneous sweating is generally ascribed to yang vacuity, while night sweating is generally ascribed to yin vacuity.

When combined appropriately, Mu Li San can be used to treat sweating from either yang vacuity or yin vacuity. It is essentially a formula that treats the branch problem of sweating, and it can be used in combination with other base formulas to treat sweating from a variety of causes. However, it is typically contraindicated in cases of sweating due to external contraction because of its astringent nature.

Yu Ping Feng San (Jade Wind–Barrier Powder)

Fang Feng (Saposhnikoviae Radix)

Huang Qi (Astragali Radix)

Bai Zhu (Atractylodis Macrocephalae Rhizoma)

Yu Ping Feng San boosts qi, secures the exterior, and checks sweating. It is a commonly used formula to treat spontaneous sweating due to exterior vacuity, and easy contraction of wind evil. Within a modular approach, Yu Ping Feng San is a useful base formula for treating a wide range of conditions where defense qi is weak; it is particularly common in treating patients who frequently suffer from conditions such as common colds and allergies.

When defense qi is weak, it is unable to secure the exterior, so the interstices are loose and empty. Construction–yin cannot be safeguarded, so the fluids discharge outwards; this causes spontaneous sweating from exterior vacuity, as well as aversion to wind and a vacuous pulse. When there is exterior vacuity and the qi is weak, the skin and hair are loose and slack. This allows for easy contraction of wind evil, causing common colds.

As in many formulas, the medicinals in Yu Ping Feng San have a relationship of complementary opposition. When Huang Qi is combined with Fang Feng, it is able to secure the exterior without retaining evil. When Fang Feng is combined with Huang Qi, it dispels evil without damaging right. This complementary opposition provides supplementation within dispersing, and dispersing within supplementation.

This formula and Gui Zhi Tang (Cinnamon Twig Decoction) both treat exterior vacuity spontaneous sweating. However, Yu Ping Feng San primarily reaches the exterior to secure the exterior and check sweating, and it primarily treats spontaneous sweating due to defense vacuity. By contrast, Gui Zhi Tang regulates construction and defense, and is used to treat spontaneous sweating due to disharmony of construction and defense. Gui Zhi Tang also resolves the exterior, so it is used to treat externally contracted wind–cold in exterior vacuity patterns.

Sheng Mai San (Pulse–Engendering Powder)

> Ren Shen (Ginseng Radix)
>
> Mai Men Dong (Ophiopogonis Radix)
>
> Wu Wei Zi (Schisandrae Fructus)

Sheng Mai San is a very useful formula for the modular approach to formula combining. It is a basic formula for treating qi and yin vacuity, and is particularly appropriate for conditions of chronic cough in cases where qi and yin have been damaged. It is also an important formula for treating fatigue, and it can be easily added to other qi–supplementing formulas such as Bu Zhong Yi Qi Tang (Center–Supplementing Qi–Boosting Decoction).

Sheng Mai San has a relatively neutral temperature because the mild warmth of Ren Shen is balanced by the cool nature of Mai Men Dong. Ren Shen supplements qi and boosts liquid while Mai Men Dong nourishes yin. All three medicinals enter the heart and quiet the spirit, and Wu Wei Zi helps to converse yin and supplement the kidney. All three medicinals also supplement the lung, making the formula particularly useful for patients with dry cough and a weak voice. Additionally, Sheng Mai San can be added to kidney–supplementing formulas such as Liu Wei Di Huang Wan (Six–Ingredient Rehmannia Pill), which creates a formula that is very similar in principle to Mai Wei Di Huang Wan (Ophiopogon and Rehmannia Pill).

Suo Quan Wan (Stream–Reducing Pill)

Wu Yao (Linderae Radix)

Yi Zhi Ren (Alpiniae Oxyphyllae Fructus)

Shan Yao (Dioscoreae Rhizoma)

Suo Quan Wan warms the kidney and dispels cold, reduces urine and checks enuresis. It is a major formula for frequent urination, as well as for enuresis in children. The combination of these three medicinals warms without drying, and eliminates vacuity cold. This allows kidney qi to be restored and reduces the frequent urination and enuresis. While the medicinal strength of this formula is mild, it can be augmented with other warming, supplementing, and securing medicinals if the condition is more severe.

Dao Chi San (Red–Abducting Powder)

Mu Tong (Akebiae Trifoliatae Caulis)

Dan Zhu Ye (Lophatheri Herba)

Sheng Di Huang (Rehmanniae Radix)

Gan Cao Shao (Glycyrrhizae Radix Tenuis)

Dao Chi San is a basic formula that frees urination to treat hot patterns of strangury (*lin*). It is a base formula that can be easily added to for a variety of problems. For example, it can be elaborated on to form more complex formulas such as Long Dan Xie Gan Tang (Gentian Liver–Draining Decoction), which contains all the medicinals in Dao Chi San except for Dan Zhu Ye.

Dao Chi San clears the heart and nourishes yin while disinhibiting water and freeing strangury. It treats patterns of exuberant heat in the heart channel. There may be vexing heat in the heart and chest, thirst and a red face, desire for cold drinks, and sores of the mouth and tongue. There may also be heart heat spreading to the small intestine, causing reddish, rough, and painful urination.

Although Dao Chi San was originally indicated for heart fire spreading to the small intestine, it can be used for a variety of patterns associated with strangury and heat. For example, Dao Chi San can be seen as a base in the formula Xiao Ji Yin Zi (Field Thistle Drink), a major formula for bloody urination (*xue lin*). Xiao Ji Yin Zi can be elaborated from Dao Chi San by adding Xiao Ji (Cirsii Herba), Ou Jie (Nelumbinis Rhizomatis Nodus), Pu Huang (Typhae Pollen), Hua Shi (Talcum), Zhi Zi (Gardeniae Fructus), and Dang Gui (Angelicae Sinensis Radix). With appropriate modifications, Dao Chi San can also be used as a base to make a formula similar to Ba Zheng San (Eight Corrections Powder) for heat strangury patterns.

Zuo Jin Wan (Left Metal Pill)

> Huang Lian (Coptidis Rhizoma)
>
> Wu Zhu Yu (Evodiae Fructus)

Zuo Jin Wan is a very small but special formula. It clears and drains liver fire, downbears counterflow and checks vomiting. As a small formula unit, it can be easily added to other prescriptions, such as Chai Hu Shu Gan San (Bupleurum Liver–Coursing Powder) or prescriptions created to harmonize the stomach and treat vomiting of acidic liquid.

Zuo Jin Wan treats liver fire invading the stomach. There may be pain in the rib–sides, "clamoring stomach" (like pain but not pain, like hunger but not hunger), acid swallowing (upflow of acid that is immediately swallowed), vomiting, bitter taste in the mouth, a red tongue with yellow fur, and a wiry rapid pulse.

This formula is used when liver depression forms fire and counterflows transversely to invade the stomach, causing liver–stomach disharmony. Inhibited qi in the liver channel causes distention and pain of the rib–sides, while liver fire invading the stomach produces the loss of the stomach's harmonious downbearing, resulting in clamoring stomach, acid swallowing, vomiting, and belching. Internal exuberance of liver fire causes the tongue and pulse presentation.

In the section on the 19 pathomechanisms, the Nei Jing states that "all counterflow upsurging is ascribed to fire," and also states that "all sour retching and vomiting…is ascribed to heat." This is the underlying theory within this formula, but the special relationship of Huang Lian (Coptidis Rhizoma) and Wu Zhu Yu (Evodiae Fructus) is its most unique feature.

Huang Lian enters the heart, liver, and stomach channels, and it directly clears liver fire. When liver fire is cleared, it no longer invades the stomach. It also drains stomach fire; when stomach fire is cleared, the stomach qi downbears on its own. Additionally, Huang Lian drains heart fire, which corresponds to the principle of "treating repletion by draining the child."

If only bitter–cold medicinals are used to treat fire depressed in the liver channel, there is a fear that the coolness will cause obstruction and make the condition difficult to resolve. Therefore, a small amount of Wu Zhu Yu is used to open liver depression and downbear stomach counterflow. Wu Zhu Yu helps Huang Lian to harmonize the stomach and check vomiting while also preventing damage to the stomach from the large quantity of bitter–cold Huang Lian. Wu Zhu Yu also helps guide Huang Lian to the liver channel, so some texts consider it to be a courier in addition to being a paradoxical assistant.

The combination of one cold and one hot medicinal in Zuo Jin Wan is very notable, and the formula has been studied extensively for many different clinical indications. Additionally, research has been done to evaluate the effects of decocting these two medicinals together, and it appears that the dosage of the two medicinals in relationship to each other affects the yield of suspected active chemical constituents. Different dose relationships of Huang Lian to Wu Zhu Yu have been recorded in Chinese medical history, but the most prominent ratio is 6 parts of Huang Lian to 1 part of Wu Zhu Yu (from Zhu Dan–Xi).

Cang Er Zi San (Xanthium Powder)

Cang Er Zi (Xanthii Fructus)

Xin Yi Hua (Magnoliae Flos)

Bai Zhi (Angelicae Dahuricae Radix)

Bo He (Menthae Herba)

Cang Er Zi San is a very useful formula for treating nasal congestion. It is particularly indicated for the TCM disease category of deep source nasal congestion (*bi yuan*), but when combined appropriately it can be used to treat many different patterns of nasal congestion.

In the original formula presentation, there may be nasal congestion and loss of the sense of smell, incessant turbid nasal mucus, and frontal headache. The combination of Cang Er Zi, Xin Yi Hua, and Bai Zhi opens the nose, while Bo He balances the warmth of the primary ingredients with its cooling nature. Bo He also helps to resolve the exterior, while Bai Zhi helps to treat frontal headache.

Cang Er Zi San treats wind–heat deep source nasal congestion. Therefore, the formula aromatically opens the orifice (of the nose) and primarily dispels wind and dissipates heat. Paradoxically, other sources indicate that the powder is taken with scallions and green tea, and the formula disperses wind–cold while freeing the orifice of the nose. In fact, some texts treat this formula as a derivative of Chuan Xiong Cha Tiao San (Tea–Blended Chuanxiong Powder), a major formula for headache in cases of external contraction.

For patterns of deep source nasal congestion caused by depressed heat in the gallbladder channel, combine Cang Er Zi San with Long Dan Xie Gan Tang (Gentian Liver–Draining Decoction). If there is exuberant liver–gallbladder fire with severe headache, constipation, reddish urine, rashness, impatience, and irascibility, consider using a modification of the formula Dang Gui Long Hui Wan (Chinese Angelica, Gentian, and Aloe Pill), which drains fire from the liver and gallbladder.

In cases of external contraction with cough, panting, and heat effusion, Cang Er Zi San may be combined with formulas such as Ma Xing Gan Shi Tang (Ephedra, Apricot Kernel, Licorice, and Gypsum Decoction). For wind–heat patterns with prominent sore throat, consider combining Cang Er Zi San with formulas such as Yin Qiao San (Lonicera and Forsythia Powder).

In cases of allergies with significant nasal congestion, Cang Er Zi San may be combined with formulas that treat the root problem, such as Yu Ping Feng San (Jade Wind–Barrier Powder) or Ren Shen Ge Jie San (Ginseng and Gecko Powder). Such formulas treat patterns associated with lung qi vacuity or lung and kidney vacuity. Cases ascribed to spleen qi vacuity can be treated by using Cang Er Zi San with formulas

such as Shen Ling Bai Zhu San (Ginseng, Poria, and White Atractylodes Powder) or Bu Zhong Yi Qi Tang (Center–Supplementing Qi–
Boosting Decoction).

For cases of nasal congestion due to depressed heat in the lung channel,
Cang Er Zi San can be modified by adding medicinals such as Huang
Qin (Scutellariae Radix) and Sang Bai Pi (Mori Cortex). Nasal conges-
tion due to damp–heat in the spleen channel can be treated by using
Cang Er Zi San with Xie Huang San (Yellow–Draining Powder).

In cases of nasal congestion with dryness, use caution when using Cang
Er Zi San so that the dryness is not exacerbated. Consider additions
such as Xing Ren (Armeniacae Semen), Chuan Bei Mu (Fritillariae Cirrhosae Bulbus), and Sang Ye (Mori Folium), or combine Cang Er Zi San
with other base formulas such as Sang Xing Tang (Mulberry Leaf and
Apricot Kernel Decoction), Qing Zao Jiu Fei Tang (Dryness–Clearing
Lung–Rescuing Decoction), or Bai He Gu Jin Tang (Lily Bulb Metal–Securing Decoction).

Gui Zhi Fu Ling Wan (Cinnamon Twig and Poria Pill)

Gui Zhi (Cinnamomi Ramulus)

Fu Ling (Poria)

Chi Shao (Paeoniae Radix Rubra)

Mu Dan Pi (Moutan Cortex)

Tao Ren (Persicae Semen)

Gui Zhi Fu Ling Wan was one of the first formulas in the history of Chinese medical gynecology, and it remains one of the most common base
formulas in gynecology today. It is traditionally used for cold–damp
and blood stasis patterns of gynecological masses, known in Chinese
medicine as *zheng jia* (concretions and conglomerations).

Gui Zhi Fu Ling Wan was first recorded in the *Jin Gui Yao Lue (Essential
Prescriptions of the Golden Coffer)*, where it was used to treat stirring fetus
in pregnant women with a history of blood stasis. It illustrates several
herbal combinations that have become standard pairs, such as the com-

bination of Chi Shao and Mu Dan Pi for blood stasis, or Gui Zhi with Fu Ling to treat patterns of dampness. The balance of cool and warm medicinals within Gui Zhi Fu Ling Wan produces a formula that is warm but not overly hot, and the formula has a good ability to quicken the blood without damaging right qi.

For cases with fixed concretions (masses due to blood stasis), E Zhu (Curcumae Rhizoma) and San Leng (Sparganii Rhizoma) may be added to Gui Zhi Fu Ling Wan. These additions are common for conditions such as uterine fibroids, which is often characterized under the TCM pattern of concretions and conglomerations (zheng jia).

In patients with significant pain due to blood stasis, common additions include the formula Shi Xiao San (Sudden Smile Powder) and the single medicinal Yan Hu Suo (Corydalis Rhizoma). Gui Zhi Fu Ling Wan can also be added to formulas such as Chai Hu Shu Gan San (Bupleurum Liver–Coursing Powder) or Jia Wei Xiao Yao San (Supplemented Free Wanderer Powder) to treat patients with liver qi depression and blood stasis.

In cases of congealing cold–damp with blood stasis, Gui Zhi Fu Ling Wan is useful because it uses the warm, freeing action of Gui Zhi in conjunction with blood–quickening medicinals. For patterns with prominent cold signs, warming agents such as Wu Zhu Yu (Evodiae Fructus), Xiao Hui Xiang (Foeniculi Fructus), and Fu Zi (Aconiti Radix Lateralis Praeparata) may be added. Alternatively, the formula Shao Fu Zhu Yu Tang (Lesser Abdomen Stasis–Expelling Decoction) may be added.

For patients with concretions and conglomerations due to phlegm–damp complicated by blood stasis, Gui Zhi Fu Ling Wan can be used with formulas such as Er Chen Tang (Two Matured Ingredients Decoction) and Xiao Luo Wan (Scrofula–Dispersing Pill).

Beyond concretions and conglomerations, Gui Zhi Fu Ling Wan can be used as a gentle and warming formula for quickening the blood in general. It stands out as a blood–moving formula because it was originally created for use in pregnancy. Overall, Gui Zhi Fu Ling Wan is quite balanced and flexible in terms of its potential applications. It can be used with various other base formulas to add a balanced, warming and blood–quickening action to the final prescription.

Additionally, adding Yi Yi Ren (Coicis Semen) to Gui Zhi Fu Ling Wan forms an empirical Japanese Kampo formula for skin diseases and acne due to blood stasis.

Xiao Luo Wan (Scrofula–Dispersing Pill)

Mu Li (Ostreae Concha)

Zhe Bei Mu (Fritillariae Thunbergii Bulbus)

Xuan Shen (Scrophulariae Radix)

Xiao Luo Wan is a formula that was originally indicated for scrofula. However, beyond its textbook indications for nodules on the neck, it can be used to soften hardness and disperse binds in a variety of applications when combined appropriately. The ability of Xiao Luo Wan to soften hardness and disperse binds can be further accentuated with the addition of medicinals such as Xia Ku Cao (Prunellae Spica), Bie Jia (Trionycis Carapax), Hai Zao (Sargassum), and Kun Bu (Laminariae/Eckloniae Thallus).

It is not uncommon for Xiao Luo Wan to be used in gynecology for conditions such as ovarian cysts or uterine fibroids in cases that are ascribed to phlegm–damp stasis. In such applications, it is often combined with formulas such as Er Chen Tang (Two Matured Ingredients Decoction) or Kai Yu Er Chen Tang (Depression–Opening Two Matured Ingredients Decoction).

Ling Gui Zhu Gan Tang (Poria, Cinnamon Twig, White Atractylodes, and Licorice Decoction)

Fu Ling (Poria)

Gui Zhi (Cinnamomi Ramulus)

Bai Zhu (Atractylodis Macrocephalae Rhizoma)

Gan Cao (Glycyrrhizae Radix)

Ling Gui Zhu Gan Tang is a formula that was originally indicated for patterns of rheum (pathological thin liquid). It utilizes a very concise and effective combination of four medicinals and offers a perfect base for elaboration in several different directions.

Within this formula, Fu Ling and Gui Zhi again combine to regulate water. Fu Ling percolates dampness and fortifies the spleen while the warm and freeing Gui Zhi promotes the qi transformation function of the bladder. Bai Zhu fortifies the spleen, dries dampness, and disinhibits water, while Gan Cao supplements the spleen and harmonizes the formula. This simple and eloquent combination can be further built for a variety of other conditions.

For yang vacuity with water swelling, Ling Gui Zhu Gan Tang can be combined with Zhen Wu Tang (True Warrior Decoction) or Shen Qi Wan (Kidney Qi Pill). Alternatively, medicinals such as Fu Zi (Aconiti Radix Lateralis Praeparata) and Ze Xie (Alismatis Rhizoma) may be added to Ling Gui Zhu Gan Tang to treat yang vacuity water swelling. For severe water swelling, the formula Wu Ling San (Poria Five Powder) can be added as well.

Ling Gui Zhu Gan Tang is also very close in nature to Li Zhong Wan (Center–Rectifying Pill) and Si Jun Zi Tang (Four Gentlemen Decoction). By adding Ren Shen (Ginseng Radix) to further supplement spleen qi and Gan Jiang (Zingiberis Rhizoma) to warm the center, Ling Gui Zhu Gan Tang can be easily modified to form a center–warming, qi–supplementing formula.

The formula Er Chen Tang (Two Matured Ingredients Decoction) can be added to Ling Gui Zhu Gan Tang to treat patients with spleen vacuity, exuberant dampness, and water swelling. Er Chen Tang dries dampness, fortifies the spleen, and harmonizes the stomach, and it can be added at varying dosage levels according to need. For patients with spleen vacuity and water swelling, Huang Qi (Astragali Radix) and Fang Ji (Stephaniae Tetrandrae Radix) may be added as well.

Zeng Ye Tang (Humor–Increasing Decoction)

Mai Men Dong (Ophiopogonis Radix)

Xuan Shen (Scrophulariae Radix)

Sheng Di Huang (Rehmanniae Radix)

Zeng Ye Tang is a very concise formula for supplementing yin and boosting liquid. It is cold in nature, and is often used to treat conditions with heat signs in the upper body (supplementing water to control fire). In particular, Xuan Shen and Sheng Di Huang clear heat and boost liquid, while Mai Men Dong clears heat and quiets the spirit.

Zeng Ye Tang is a perfect building block for formula combining. On its own, it is a useful intestine–moistening formula to treat constipation due to yin vacuity and liquid damage. It is also well–suited to treating the aftermath of febrile disease in cases where yin and fluids have been damaged by heat. Zeng Ye Tang is an important formula to consider in warm disease, and it can be used as a base to build more complex warm disease formulas, such as Qing Ying Tang (Construction–Clearing Decoction).

For more severe constipation in patients that does not respond to Zeng Ye Tang, Da Huang (Rhei Radix et Rhizoma) and Mang Xiao (Natrii Sulfas) can be added. This combination forms the formula Zeng Ye Cheng Qi Tang (Humor–Increasing Qi–Coordinating Decoction), which is a representative formula for the principle of simultaneous supplementing and attacking therapy. It is used for yang brightness (yang ming) disease with constipation due to damage to the fluids, when neither precipitation nor enriching yin liquid and increasing humor is effective.

When combined appropriately, Zeng Ye Tang can be used for a wide range of conditions associated with yin vacuity and heat. Regardless of whether it is used in large doses as a principle formula or whether it is used in small doses as an auxiliary formula, Zeng Ye Tang has an important place in formula combining.

Additionally, Zeng Ye Tang can be used as a modification in formulas to treat sore throat, especially in cases of yin vacuity with internal heat. For cases of thirst and severe sore throat due to fire–toxin, Zeng Ye Tang can be used in combination with medicinals such as Ban Lan Gen (Isatidis Radix), Huang Qin (Scutellariae Radix), Niu Bang Zi (Arctii Fructus), and She Gan (Belamcandae Rhizoma).

Suan Zao Ren Tang (Spiny Jujube Decoction)

> Suan Zao Ren (Ziziphi Spinosi Semen)
>
> Fu Ling (Poria)
>
> Zhi Mu (Anemarrhenae Rhizoma)
>
> Chuan Xiong (Chuanxiong Rhizoma)
>
> Gan Cao (Glycyrrhizae Radix)

Suan Zao Ren Tang represents a very nice unit for formula combining. It nourishes the blood and quiets the spirit, and also clears heat and eliminates vexation. It can be used to add a nourishing, spirit–quieting aspect to a compound prescription, and it can be further elaborated to treat vacuity insomnia from a variety of causes.

Suan Zao Ren Tang also has a slight ability to check sweating, and Wu Wei Zi (Schisandrae Fructus) and Ma Huang Gen (Ephedrae Radix) can be added to treat night sweating. For palpitations, Long Chi (Mastodi Dentis Fossilia) and Long Yan Rou (Longan Arillus) can be added to Suan Zao Ren Tang.

Gan Mai Da Zao Tang (Licorice, Wheat, and Jujube Decoction)

> Xiao Mai (Tritici Fructus)
>
> Da Zao (Jujubae Fructus)
>
> Gan Cao (Glycyrrhizae Radix)

The formula Gan Mai Da Zao Tang was originally created to treat a disease in women known as visceral agitation, though it is now used for both genders. Typical manifestations of visceral agitation include disturbed emotions, sorrow and crying without reason, frequent stretching and yawning, and mental fatigue. It is know generally thought that visceral agitation is caused by emotions causing liver depression transforming into fire, which damages yin and results in dual vacuity of the spleen and heart.

Gan Mai Da Zao Tang is a balanced, gentle formula. It nourishes the heart and quiets the spirit, and harmonizes the center and supplements spleen qi. The simplicity and gentle nourishing nature of this formula makes it applicable for a wide range of applications in formula combining.

Challenges in Formula Combining

There are a few features of the formula combining method that pose logistical challenges and unresolved questions. Formula combining allows one to add medicinals but not to subtract them, so there are often ingredients present that could be eliminated if multiple formulas are compounded together.

There are many approaches to formula combining. The basic outline of treatment ideas suggested in this chapter represents just the tip of the iceberg. At the beginning, it is easiest to start with relatively small, simple formulas that have clear principles and few ingredients. This approach is also ideal for practitioners that maintain small pharmacies or new practitioners that want to start a dynamic pharmacy with minimal overhead. However, formula combining can get much more complicated than the basic approaches outlined here.

In Taiwan, formula combining is extremely common, and practitioners routinely use 2–4 formulas together in any given prescription. Chinese medical doctors in Taiwan memorize hundreds of classical formulas, and any given pharmacy has hundreds of classical formulas on the shelf to choose from. Consequently, Taiwanese doctors tend to prescribe relatively complex blends of even fairly large formulas, resulting in a very distinctive prescription style that takes time to learn and appreciate.

The widespread use of both raw herbs and granules in Taiwan has made Taiwan a unique environment for formula combining. The traditional method of raw herb decoctions remains common in Taiwan, so Chinese medical doctors there regularly use two independent systems of formulation, one for granules (covered by insurance) and one for raw herbs (not covered by insurance).

By contrast, doctors from mainland China are accustomed to writing raw herb prescriptions only. In mainland China, the main revolution of convenience revolved around the use of small decoction machines, and granules are a relatively late arrival. In comparison to Taiwan, mainstream pharmacies in China have relatively few unmodified classical formulas. Most mainland Chinese prepared medicines are custom formulations and proprietary mixtures rather than classical formulas in granule form, so the marketplace availability varies significantly between the two regions.

Granule use has now begun to take off in mainland China, but the primary products available are single herb extracts. Compound classical granule formulas remain rare on the Chinese domestic granule market (at least in hospitals and large clinics), so there has not been a major change in the prescription style on the mainland as there has been in Taiwan. Consequently, Chinese medical doctors who move to Taiwan from mainland China often have a difficult time accepting the Taiwanese method of compounding whole formulas.

The fact that additions can be made but removing ingredients is not possible results in some final compound formulas that contain 40 ingredients or more. This fact causes some people to view formula compounding as too chaotic, because some medicinals overlap in multiple formulas and some unnecessary medicinals are present in the final prescription. However, whole formulas can also be thought of as representing a clear, single principle so there is some inherent validity in the formula combining approach. After decades of use of both methods, it is clear that both approaches can achieve satisfactory clinic results.

One challenge to be aware of is the duplication of ingredients when multiple formulas are combined. If several formulas have the same ingredient, an item that was originally intended as an auxiliary medicinal can ultimately be given at a dose that is higher than that of some of the more important medicinals. The most common example of this problem is Gan Cao, which appears in many formulas. If several formulas that contain Gan Cao are combined, the relative dosage of Gan Cao can move from that of a courier to that of a sovereign medicinal. Thus, it is important to have a strong command of formula ingredients to minimize the problem of duplication. In some situations, duplication may be desirable to add emphasis to a certain principle, but in other situations duplication of medicinals can upset the balance of the formula.

Case Studies

Case1:

A 26 year–old male presented with an acute episode of ulcerative colitis. He had suffered from periodic episodes of ulcerative colitis several times over the past few years, and often required hospitalization and IV prednisone to control the severe bleeding and diarrhea. In this particular episode, he presented with watery bowel movements characterized by blood and mucus (approximately 20 times per day), accompanied by tenesmus. At the time of examination, he appeared fatigued from the prolonged diarrhea and was anxious about the possibility of hospitalization if the condition did not improve. He associates the condition with significant emotional stress and presented with abdominal distention, poor appetite, a puffy pale tongue with thick greasy yellow fur and a bowstring, slippery pulse. After questioning, he was diagnosed with the Chinese medical disease category of dysentery (痢疾), presenting with a pattern of liver depression and spleen vacuity complicated by dampness and heat.

The first prescription was based on Si Ni San (Counterflow Cold Powder) plus Tong Xie Yao Fang (Important Formula for Painful Diarrhea), with the addition of heat–clearing and dampness–drying herbs.

Prescription #1:

> Si Ni San (Counterflow Cold Powder) 5g
>
> Tong Xie Yao Fang (Important Formula for Painful Diarrhea) 5g
>
> Huang Lian (Coptidis Rhizoma) 1g
>
> Mu Xiang (Aucklandiae Radix) 1g
>
> Bai Jiang Cao (Patriniae Herba) 1g
>
> Hong Teng (Sargentodoxae Caulis) 1g
>
> Chen Pi (Citri Reticulatae Pericarpium) 0.8g

Qin Pi (Fraxini Cortex) 1g

Yi Yi Ren (Coicis Semen) [dry–fried] 1.2g

Huang Bai (Phellodendri Cortex) 1g

This prescription was given for three days, at which point the tenesmus, bleeding, and mucus had improved markedly. The frequency of bowel movements was reduced dramatically but the patient still had watery diarrhea with blood. The tongue fur was less yellow and greasy and the chief compliant now centered on fatigue and diarrhea. The prescription was modified as follows.

Prescription #2:

Si Ni San (Counterflow Cold Powder) 4g

Tong Xie Yao Fang (Important Formula for Painful Diarrhea) 4g

Huang Lian (Coptidis Rhizoma) 1g

Mu Xiang (Aucklandiae Radix) 1g

Chen Pi (Citri Reticulatae Pericarpium) 1g

Yi Yi Ren (Coicis Semen) [dry–fried] 1.5g

Huang Bai (Phellodendri Cortex) 1g

Fu Ling (Poria) 1.5g

Shan Yao (Dioscoreae Rhizoma) 1.5g

Ren Shen (Ginseng Radix) 1g

Qian Shi (Euryales Semen) 1.5g

Xian He Cao (Agrimoniae Herba) 1g

Following six days of this formula, the patient continued to have improvement in the frequency of the diarrhea and the bleeding continued to reduce. The tenesmus and mucus were resolved and the patient was now able to consume solid food without provoking the diarrhea. Bowel movements remained watery but were limited to a few times per day. The formula was modified to strengthen the spleen and astringent medicinals were added.

Prescription #3:

Si Ni San (Counterflow Cold Powder) 5g

Shen Ling Bai Zhu San (Ginseng, Poria, and White Atractylodes Powder) 7g

Xian He Cao (Agrimoniae Herba) 1g

Chen Pi (Citri Reticulatae Pericarpium) 1g

He Zi (Chebulae Fructus) 1g

Wu Mei (Fructus Mume) 1g

Variations of this formula were given for 14 days, with consistent improvement that eventually led to complete resolution.

Case 2:

A 47 year–old woman presents with an enlarged uterus due to uterine fibroids and heavy menstrual bleeding. Her uterus is slightly visible through her clothing and its superior and lateral borders can be clearly palpated. Her chief complaint is her appearance (she is self-conscious about her belly), but she acknowledges that she feels fatigue after her period, which is regular, lasts 8–12 days and is characterized by thick, dark blood with many large clots. She also complains of dizziness, poor concentration and memory, and poor appetite. Her pulse is thin and weak, and her tongue is pale–purple with distended sublingual veins. Based on a Chinese medical diagnosis of profuse menstruation manifesting with a pattern of qi and blood vacuity and blood stasis, the following granule prescription was given:

Gui Zhi Fu Ling Wan (Cinnamon Twig and Poria Pill) 5g

Gui Pi Tang (Spleen–Returning Decoction) g

San Leng (Sparganii Rhizoma) 1g

E Zhu (Curcumae Rhizoma) 1g

Yi Mu Cao (Leonuri Herba) 1g

Alternatively, the following prescription could be made by combining singles instead of using base formulas:

Huang Qi (Astragali Radix) 2g

Dang Gui (Angelicae Sinensis Radix) 1g

Bai Zhu (Atractylodis Macrocephalae Rhizoma) 1.2g

Fu Ling (Poria) 2g

Ren Shen (Ginseng Radix) 0.8g

Bai Shao (Paeoniae Radix Alba) 1.5g

Tao Ren (Persicae Semen) 1.2g

Chi Shao (Paeoniae Radix Rubra) 1g

Mu Dan Pi (Moutan Cortex) 0.8g

E Zhu (Curcumae Rhizoma) 1.2g

San Leng (Sparganii Rhizoma) 1.2g

Yi Mu Cao (Leonuri Herba) 1g

Zhi Gan Cao (Glycyrrhizae Radix Praeparata) 0.5g

During episodes of heavy menstruation, Yi Mu Cao, San Leng, E Zhu, and perhaps Tao Ren, Chi Shao, and/or Mu Dan Pi should be removed, and medicinals such as Pu Huang (Typhae Pollen), Qian Cao (Rubiae Radix), San Qi (Notoginseng Radix) and Hai Piao Xiao (Sepiae Endoconcha) may be added.

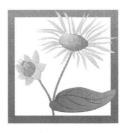

CHAPTER SEVEN

Setting Up a Granule Pharmacy

How to Assess Granule Products

Assessing the quality of crude herbs requires a significant degree of specialized skill. Different regions use different techniques to cut and process medicinals, so practitioners need to be familiar with multiple forms of the same medicinal before grading and quality assessment becomes possible. By contrast, in granule form the appearance of each item is generally the same except for its color and aroma. Thus, there is a bit of a learning curve when it comes to knowing what to look for in granules.

To start, look at the gross texture of the granule. Is it a fine powder or a coarse, large kernel granule? Neither form is necessarily better than the other, but they tend to use different excipients. The amount of excipient varies from one product to the next and from one brand to the next, and each excipient has its own unique advantages and disadvantages (for example, dextrin dissolves better than starch but it tends to absorb moisture more quickly in hot, humid environments). For most substances, inert excipients should be minimized as long as the product does not clump upon exposure to air.

As mentioned previously, fine powders are often preferable if the patient takes the powder directly by mouth. Most of the granules that are made in Taiwan and Japan fall into this category. The manufacturing approach in Taiwan and Japan typically yields a product that does not clump easily, but relatively high proportions of starch (around 35–50%) are often used because fine powders tend to clump easily if there is an inadequate amount of excipient. Fine powders have more surface area and often have a stronger fragrance than coarse granules when the bottle is first opened.

Coarse granules can often achieve a higher concentration than fine powders without clumping together. However, coarse granules perform best when dissolved in hot water, so they are not as good for patients that eat the powder directly without dissolving it first. Coarse granules tend to have a milder fragrance in their dry state than fine granules because they have less surface area.

To test granules for quality, get more than one brand and test them side–by–side. Naturally, a full lab is better than the naked senses because constituent levels can be assessed. Most people do not have access to analytical equipment, so taste, smell, and perceived efficacy are the main parameters that most practitioners use to assess quality.

To start, open the bottles and smell the powder. It should smell clean and any aromatic herbs will tend to have a deep fragrance. Next, boil water and dissolve a weighed amount of granules from each brand into a different cup with the same volume of water. It is important to use a scale instead of a spoon because different granules vary significantly in their density. If one measures by volume instead of weight, one spoonful of large granules will weigh more than the same spoonful of fine powder.

Pay attention to the dissolution time. The whole product should dissolve within a few minutes of stirring in freshly boiled water. Next, let it sit and cool for a few minutes. If powdery sediment precipitates out of the solution, the carrier used is most likely starch or raw herb powder. The amount of starch at the bottom of the cup may vary from one brand to another, and some brands may have no sediment at all. Patients that take granules by dissolving them in water generally prefer granules that dissolve completely.

After checking the dissolution, do a taste test to assess the flavor. The flavor should be deep and rich, just like a decoction. Pay attention to whether your palate can detect distinctive flavors of individual substances such as Mu Dan Pi (Moutan Cortex), Dang Gui (Angelicae Sinensis Radix), or Ren Shen (Ginseng Radix). The more the flavor and color resembles a decoction, the better. There should be a slight fragrance to the steam coming off the cup, indicating that the essential oils are intact. Distinctive flavors should come through—one should be able to taste the individual ingredients rather than just tasting one indistinct, uniform flavor. The flavor should be vibrant and dynamic, not bland or unpleasant.

Compounding Granules and the FDA

U.S. FDA law currently regards granules as dietary supplements. In the U.S., specific laws regarding cGMPs (current Good Manufacturing Practices) apply to dietary supplements, and many practitioners are uncertain about the degree to which these laws affect their compounding practices. While there are fundamentally some gray areas in the law, it is good for practitioners to be aware of the general scope of these new laws and their impact on herbal pharmacies.

The FDA's cGMP laws primarily revolve around maintaining good records and clean, safe manufacturing practices. While the laws are primarily focused on manufacturers, individual compounding facilities technically do not have an absolute exemption from cGMPs. In general, the FDA has stated that they will exercise "discretionary enforcement" for licensed practitioners that see patients on a one–on–one basis. In other words, minimal enforcement is expected as long as a trained professional sees a patient individually and prepares medicine that is customized for their case. Enforcement discretion does not apply to clinics that prepare medicine in large batches and dispense products to customers that have not had any individual evaluation.

In terms of dietary supplements and GMP law, different regulatory tiers apply to companies that simply "hold" sealed bottles rather than companies that "manufacture" products. The responsibilities of companies that hold products (such as a retailer that stocks sealed bottles on the shelves) are much less complicated than the responsibilities that apply to manufacturing. In other words, selling sealed bottles

Technically, any time the sealed bottles are broken and individual ingredients are compounded together the FDA regulates the company as a "manufacturer." This creates a gray area because most individual practitioners and clinics do open bottles and compound products together, but they tend to see patients on a one–on–one basis and thus fall under discretionary enforcement. The rub is that despite the FDA's official statement that discretionary enforcement applies to individual practitioners, technically the scope of the law clearly regards compounding of custom formulas as "manufacturing" (thus subject to cGMP rules).

Achieving true cGMP–level compliance is unrealistic for most small businesses and compounding pharmacies. Compliance requires the management of a host of complex details and requires a facility that contains an appropriate configuration of sinks, surfaces, entrances, temperature control, etc. The cost of setting up and maintaining such a facility generally runs into tens if not hundreds of thousands of dollars, so very few Chinese medical dispensaries are able to reach cGMP compliance. Such pharmacies tend to rely on the provision for "discretionary enforcement," and in most circumstances the risk of problems is quite low if the clinic is well–managed. Unfortunately, there is a fear that enforcement discretion could go out the window if a true adverse event and associated lawsuits arose, so many clinics choose to be as vigilant as possible when it comes to safe compounding practices and well–organized recordkeeping.

Setting Up

When it comes to setting up a granule pharmacy, the first step is to start with a reliable supplier. There are multiple quality granule producers to choose from, and choosing a good source will save significant effort later. As mentioned above, assessing the quality of the product itself is essential. Beyond choosing the right product in terms of quality, consistency, and value, it is also important to assess your supplier on the basis of GMP issues.

A supplier that runs a tight ship with their own GMP management is well–positioned to offer support when it comes to helping your clinic maintain good records. While there is general consensus that true GMP compliance is beyond the reach of the average clinic, maintaining a good paper trail and being informed and proactive about safety issues will ultimately be very beneficial in the unlikely event that FDA issues ever arise. Below are some of the basic things to keep in mind:

Choosing a Supplier

As required by law, GMP–certified manufacturers have safeguards in place to track their inventory, manage recalls, record adverse events, etc. All the key factories that produce granules have GMP–certification in their home country, yet some factories have far more wide–reaching efforts than others when it comes to meeting international regulations. For example, some factories have only local GMP certification while others also have Australian TGA certification or third–party certificated U.S. FDA cGMP certification.

There is also significant variation in the complexity and number of tests that individual manufacturers employ. For example, some companies test for only three pesticides while others test for 150 or more. Some labs use equipment that tests ppm (parts per million) while others test with equipment that can register ppb (parts per billion), so even the specified detection limit for the tests can vary. Some companies use only in–house testing while others combine in–house testing with independent third–party testing.

Testing for things like pesticides, constituents, and heavy metals can be quite expensive, and the house standards can vary significantly. For example, companies often set internal standards for heavy metals based on the national standards that correspond to their target market, and the allowance for various heavy metals varies between countries such as China, Japan, and Germany. This means that different companies may have different acceptable limits when it comes to testing results, and sometimes even the same company has requirements that vary depending on what market they are servicing with a particular product.

When choosing a supplier, it is also good to assess the degree of transparency that they provide. Do they use ethanol in their extractions or water only? Do they capture and reintroduce essential oils? Are the excipients (starch, dextrin, etc.) and concentration ratios disclosed on the label? Are certificates of analysis or testing results available upon request? Can the company track the lot numbers of your orders or is this something that needs to be done manually by the clinic? Most importantly, is the company accessible and forthcoming with information or is it difficult to find the answers that you need?

Documenting Procedures

Beyond having adequate facilities and training, true GMP compliance is characterized by extensive records that document Standard Operating Procedures (SOPs) for virtually every task that is undertaken. Despite the fact that small pharmacies do not have the resources for true GMP compliance, it is possible for a pharmacy to maintain effective SOPs that document the tasks and procedures that fit their needs. If documentation is present that specifies procedures and their implementation, the clinic will appear rigorous and vigilant to an inspector in the unlikely event that the clinic is audited by the FDA (this would typically be unexpected for small clinics unless adverse events or poor business practices are reported). While no one truly knows to what degree good SOPs will protect a small business that cannot be truly GMP compliant, the general consensus is that strong SOPs will leave a favorable impression and help to minimize problems.

When designing SOPs, one should try to cover all the minute details. What is the task, who performs it, when do they perform it, what action should be taken if a problem arises? SOPs should be made for all the different tasks that the clinic performs. Someone should sign off when they receive the shipment and they should log the lot number. It doesn't matter whether the system is high–tech or just handwritten on paper, but there should be a paper trail that allows each batch of herbs to be tracked to the patients that received them. The lot numbers should be recorded when the shipment comes in, and a system should be developed to follow who received herbs from that particular lot. If something goes wrong (product recall, broken glass jar in the clinic, etc.), a procedure should be documented to fix it. The successful resolution of the problem should be documented as well.

SOPs should also be established for things like routine maintenance and cleaning. Who sweeps the floors and how often do they do it? What steps are taken to minimize pests such as insects or rodents? Are employees required to wear clean uniforms, gloves, etc? All these details should ideally be documented, even if the details seem like common sense. For example, employees should generally be prohibited from eating in the compounding space and the herbs should not be stored on the floor. Most clinics do have such rules but often there may be no documentation that these rules exist and are followed. Vigilance when it comes to establishing compounding procedures means identifying these issues, writing SOPs, and maintaining logs that show that the SOPs are being used.

Equipment

Generally speaking, a good workspace is required. Most practitioners use a large container to mix the granules together, and this container should be cleaned in between prescriptions. A scale that is accurate to 1/10 of a gram should be used, and an SOP should be created to periodically calibrate the scale to verify its accuracy. True GMP facilities often take the extra step of having a method to check and log that the correct herbs were selected and the correct amount was weighed, but many small private clinics do not go this far.

Beyond the shelves, the workspace, and the scale, little equipment is required for a granule pharmacy. A good method of mixing the ingredients together in formulas is necessary, and there should be enough space in the mixing container to ensure that the formula is mixed adequately.

Designing Labels

According to FDA law, all products should be labeled. The FDA website itself (www.fda.gov) offers the most comprehensive guidelines for U.S. labeling laws, and similar guidelines exist for the labeling requirements in other countries. Labeling requirements are detailed and are beyond the scope of this book, but a few general guidelines are noted below.

In the U.S., granules are classified as dietary supplements. Technically, their labels require a "principle display panel" that contains the identity of the product; this label is the center panel that faces the consumer. English is the preferred language when it comes to name of the product and its ingredients, and the ingredient list should be included in the panel to the right of the principal display panel. A box titled Supplement Facts must be located to the right of the principal display panel, and the FDA publishes very precise guidelines regarding font size, bold text, the lines within the box, etc. Any other (inert) ingredients must also be listed and precise dosage directions should be included.

A few other general pieces of information are also required for proper labeling, including the name and address of the supplier, the country of origin, the net weight, and other details. Many detailed resources exist for researching this information, but the "take–home message" is that including a label on the products that are being dispensed is generally something that advocates of safe compounding guidelines universally endorse.

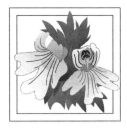

Conclusion

As a novel delivery form, granules offer some unique advantages. Convenience, portability, and safety are some of the key factors that account for the appeal of granules in the modern world, and granules often represent the most cost effective way of giving decoction–strength doses to patients that are unable or unwilling to cook raw herbs. Consequently, granules have gradually come to rival the traditional decoction as the most prominent delivery form for Chinese medicine in many countries.

The worldwide consumption of granules is truly astounding in scale. For example, research conducted by Prof. Chang Hsien–Cheh of China Medical University has demonstrated that patients in the national healthcare system in Taiwan alone consumed nearly 2.7 million kilograms of granules over a recent two–year period. Granules are prescribed in approximately 30 million patient visits in Taiwan annually by over 4,000 Chinese medical doctors. Taiwan's most widely prescribed formula, Jia Wei Xiao Yao San (Supplemented Free Wanderer Powder), accounted for a stunning 3.2% of this total. Taiwan alone consumed a mind–blowing 86.3 metric tons of Jia Wei Xiao Yao San within the two–year period between 2002 and 2003.

Entirely new prescribing styles have evolved around granules in places like Taiwan, and granules are quickly becoming the most popular delivery form in Western countries that are new to Chinese medicine. Clearly one could safely say that granules represent a revolutionary addition to the arsenal of Chinese medicine. Many practitioners swear by granules and there is a general consensus that they produce reliable clinical results. Nonetheless, despite their popularity and widespread use, granules are not universally endorsed or well–understood across the Chinese medical community.

It is always important to consider the relative merits and drawbacks to any new delivery system based on a rational assessment. Opinions on topics such as granules are influenced by many factors and cultural attitudes toward granules from region to region. Furthermore, significant variation in dosage and prescribing trends can be found in different regions, making it impossible to have one universal frame of reference. Regardless of regional style, most practitioners tend to recognize several distinct pros and cons when it comes to assessing granules.

Advantages

Convenience is one of the greatest motivating factors for many practitioners when they choose granule products. In addition to saving patients considerable time and effort, granules minimize the risk of patient error when it comes to cooking the medicinals correctly at home. Granules are far more portable and convenient than raw herbs, so compliance tends to improve without any major reduction in dosage or potency. The improved compliance yields enhanced clinical results, which is an advantage to both patients and practitioners alike.

From the perspective of the practitioner, granules offer convenience that goes unnoticed by the patient. Granules take up less space in the clinic and are easier to track when it comes to issues such as inventory control and regulatory compliance. They are more stable than raw herbs and offer better shelf life without nuisances such as insect infestation and spoilage. Generally speaking, the GMP factories that produce granules are well–equipped when it comes to ensuring that the raw herbs are correctly identified and processed, so less specialty expertise in the pharmacy is required of the dispensing practitioner. These aspects of quality control are usually combined with lot-tracing and testing for microbial contamination, heavy metals, and pesticide residues by granule factories, which further makes granules a comfortable choice for many practitioners.

Beyond safety and convenience, granules are often a good choice in terms of potency. Assuming that the supplier provides clear information on the concentration ratio, it is relatively easy to calculate a granule dose that delivers about the same amount of medicine. Furthermore, the price tends to be reasonable because granule manufacturers tend to start from whole, unsliced raw herbs and they achieve enough economy of scale to make the finished product similar in price to raw herbs.

In places such as Taiwan and Japan, granules have had a major impact on the healthcare system. The safety controls during manufacturing and the traceability of granules by batch allows for uniform regulations and improved management in regions where granule use is widespread. Additionally, large batches of granules have a degree of uniform consistency that is difficult to match with raw herbs, making granules ideal for research studies.

Disadvantages

Despite the many positive benefits of using granules, there are some practitioners that still prefer to use raw herbs. For example, Taiwan uses granules in approximately 30 million patient visits per year, and granules are the only form of herbal medicine that is reimbursed by the insurance system there. Many doctors in Taiwan feel that granules are ideal in prolonged, chronic cases that benefit from the convenience and reduced cost associated with granules. However, when it comes to severe, acute conditions, most doctors in Taiwan still believe that raw herbs are faster and stronger than granules.

It is difficult to assess whether the common Taiwanese perception that granules are milder and slower than raw herbs is based on differences in dosage or simply differences between the two delivery forms. The insurance coverage for granules in Taiwan only applies to a typical dose of about 18 grams per day, which is somewhat lower than the equivalent dose that would be prescribed if the patient took raw herbs. Thus, assessing the validity of this perspective is challenging because there are two variables present: a different delivery form as well as a different dose level.

The fact that Chinese medicine is generally a conservative field when it comes to new ideas also influences the perception of granules. Ideas change slowly and true consensus on new theories can take centuries to develop in Chinese medicine. Any new delivery system is certain to have its share of skeptics, and many older doctors in places like mainland China have been slow to warm up to granules. In some situations, it can be difficult to ascertain whether this resistance is due to a general hesitation to adopt new methods or whether the resistance is due to bona fide clinical concerns.

On the whole, the perception of granules varies significantly from place to place. The scope of products on the market tends to affect the perception of granules, and places that have had granules for a long time tend to use them more widely than places that have only started using them recently. For example, in Taiwan granules have been used for over 40 years and their acceptance is quite high. By contrast, in mainland China granules are a newer delivery system that has not penetrated the healthcare system as deeply. Granules are less common in mainland China and tend to be prevalent only in large hospitals, so the acceptance and rate of use there is lower.

The chief disadvantage of granules is the fact that the medicinals are often not cooked together. When making a formula from scratch, the easiest way to replicate a raw herb prescription is to combine single herb extracts. However, this method lacks the interaction of the herbs as they cook together in the pot. While this method is very common in the West and mainland China, some practitioners are uncomfortable with the fact that the mixed granules haven't been decocted together. Lack of interaction of the medicinals during the cooking process is thus one of the major downsides when it comes to the prescribing style of mixing single granules.

On the other hand, if one uses whole formulas that have been cooked together, a challenge arises because unnecessary ingredients cannot be removed and some items can be potentially duplicated. The compounding of whole formulas together is particularly common in Taiwan, and the conundrum posed by duplication of ingredients and inclusion of unnecessary items is one of the major shortcomings of the Taiwanese method.

Each of the approaches above has positive and negative elements and it is impossible to declare that one method is universally superior. Ultimately, people tend to use whatever style they were trained in. Unfortunately, very little in the way of training exists at present when it comes to granules. Prolonged clinical residency and internships offer doctors in Asia the opportunity to gain experience, but even in the Chinese world there are few strong academic sources that could serve as a granule handbook.

The regional variation in granule use makes the subject even more difficult to learn. Many of the influential herbal medicine teachers in the West were trained in mainland China decades ago, before granules were widely used. Such teachers may not have extensive experience with granules and many have had minimal exposure to different prescribing styles. Complicating the problem, practitioners in areas of heavy granule use such as Taiwan tend to have complex, opaque styles that are difficult to learn and are poorly elucidated in written teaching materials, and few Western practitioners have studied the Taiwanese prescribing method in detail.

The Future of Granules in the West

In the West, convenience has caused granules to be one of the most popular delivery forms of Chinese herbal medicine. Western practitioners tend to use a hybrid approach that has features of both the mainland Chinese prescribing style (building a formula from singles) and the Taiwanese prescribing style (using base formulas that have been cooked together). However, Western practitioners are often unclear about issues of dosage and concentration, and many practitioners have not been exposed to the complex variation in prescribing methods seen in Asia.

To a certain extent, the academic development of granules worldwide suffers from a similar weakness—many of the top experts on granules are somehow tied to the industry itself. Making granules is an art and a science, and most of the research and innovation happens within the private industry and is not widely shared amongst competitors. There are few academic outlets for granule experts outside the realm of chemistry, and many of the most knowledgeable people in the field tend to be employed in the private sector. Thus, our best resources for learning about the granule products are often the people that work with the companies themselves. This lends itself to a certain degree of natural bias, and makes definitive answers for many technical questions somewhat elusive.

Fundamentally, the confusion about dosage in the West is related to the fact that our primary reference for dosage information is often the vendors themselves. Many suppliers do not list the quantity of inert ingredients such as starch or dextrin, and often the concentration ratio is not provided. This makes it difficult to assess the potency of the product and its relationship to a raw herb decoction, which causes uncertainty about proper dosage. While some manufacturers publish information on the concentration ratio and try to educate the community about prescription styles and dosage calculation, practitioners often hear wildly different dosage recommendations depending on which teachers or manufacturers they talk to.

Beyond uncertainty about dosage, Western practitioners are often unaware of the tremendous variety of approaches to making granule formulas. Some practitioners prefer combining whole formulas while others prefer to build from single ingredients, but few practitioners are aware of the roots of these trends in Asia. All too often, we acquire the bias of our teachers and seldom explore alternative methods, and precious few students are bringing back cutting edge material on granules from the East.

At present, granule prescription styles and manufacturing methods are not harmonized, and a truly mature understanding of granules is not yet a global reality. There is a lot of room for progress in terms of academic exchange and development in Asian countries, and it will take time for all of this knowledge to reach the West. Ultimately, a sophisticated understanding of granules in the West will require greater academic exchange with experts in Asia, and it will require a rigorous level of investigation that is far beyond the scope of a small introductory book such as this one.

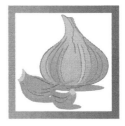

Glossary

1. Full-spectrum Extract

In the context of Chinese medicine, full-spectrum extracts tend to refer to products that reflect the natural constituent yield that is obtained from a traditional water decoction. Historically, most prescriptions have been prepared as a water decoction, so replicating a decoction is thought to provide the best approximation of the spectrum of constituents that Chinese medicine's time–tested results are based upon.

From the perspective of plant chemistry in general, one could argue that a truly full–spectrum extract would include both alcohol– and water–soluble constituents. However, only a minority of Chinese medicine's herbal products were traditionally extracted with alcohol, so the use of alcohol and other solvents is considered to introduce a variable that was not historically present for most items. Consequently, the term "full–spectrum extract" in Chinese medicine usually refers to a water–based extract that does not focus on concentrating any one single constituent, but rather focuses on concentrating all the water–soluble material in a substance without affecting the natural ratio of these constituents.

This stands in contradistinction to "standardized extracts," which tend to focus on specific constituents rather than focusing on a broad spectrum of substances that are all soluble in water. Items that are best suited to full–spectrum water extracts include medicinals that were traditionally prepared as a decoction, and medicinals that have numerous active ingredients and/or unknown active ingredients.

Many of the substances in Chinese medicine have multiple active ingredients and many others have active ingredients that are poorly understood; for some substances, no active ingredients have yet been identified. In order to preserve the diversity of constituents and the natural variation inherent in plant products, many users choose to use full–spectrum extracts because such extracts are comparable to the decoction that a patient would take if they boiled the herbs at home. We do not know which constituents or interactions between constituents are responsible for most of the effects observed with the use of Chinese herbal medicines, so it is prudent to use full–spectrum extracts as much as possible.

Full–spectrum extracts tend to leave the natural ratios of constituents intact, whereas standardized extracts focus on concentrating individual constituents or groups of constituents. It is quite likely that some of the effects that we observe are due to constituents or interactions between constituents that have not yet been adequately explored, so using extracts that focus on specific compounds at the exclusion of others introduces an unknown variable in many situations.

While most Chinese herbal medicines were traditionally used by decoction, there are a few items that were traditionally extracted with wine. For example, the medicinal Rou Cong Rong (Cistanches Herba) was historically used in alcohol extracts as well as water decoctions. It is now known that Rou Cong Rong contains active constituents that are soluble in alcohol but are not very soluble in water; consequently, full–spectrum extracts of items such as Rou Cong Rong often incorporate ethanol. Such items are generally an exception to the rule, and the term "full–spectrum extract" in Chinese medicine most commonly refers only to the concentrated extract obtained by a water decoction.

When making a full–spectrum extract, chemical testing is sometimes used to assess the potency of the product, but the goal differs from a standardized extract. For example, a company that makes a full–spectrum extract of ginseng may measure the ginsenoside content of both the raw material and the finished product. For the sake of illustration, let us assume that the company's standard for the raw material specified that the crude ginseng roots must contain a minimum of 7% ginsenosides in order to be considered acceptable. This means that the company would accept any ginseng that contained 7% ginsenosides or more. If that company then made a full–spectrum 3:1 extract, they could expect that the extract would contain at least 21% ginsenosides, and they might test to confirm that this minimum level was attained. However, the final extract could contain 22–25% ginsenosides or more, depending on the potency of the starting material. By contrast, a "standardized extract" of 21% ginsenosides would be expected to contain exactly 21%, no more, no less, and the product could be made with whatever amount of whatever quality raw material it took to achieve this 21% target.

2. Standardized Extract

Standardized extracts are produced by concentrating specific constituents so that these constituents are present at an even level from batch to batch. While a full–spectrum extract may vary from batch to batch (for example, one batch might contain 21% ginsenosides and the next might contain 24%), the standardized product would be consistently 21% every time. It might take a different amount of starting material to reach this target from batch to batch, but the final concentration of the chosen constituents would remain the same in each batch of the standardized extract. This stands in contradistinction to a full–spectrum extract that used the same amount of starting material for each batch, but obtained a different constituent yield from batch to batch because of the natural variability in the potency of the raw herbs.

A standardized extract is not very well–suited to products that have unknown active constituents, because it is not obvious which compounds the product should be standardized to in such circumstances. However, standardized extracts are ideal for substances that have well–characterized active ingredients, especially if there is high variability in the natural potency of the starting material. For example, an extract of a toxic product like datura flower would be potentially dangerous as a full–spectrum extract because one batch could contain 1% atropine while the next batch could contain 3% atropine. In the case of datura flower, the toxic but medicinal constituents atropine and scopolamine are very well–characterized scientifically. There is consensus that they are the principle active constituents, and safe use is only possible if these constituents are given at a consistent, predictable dosage. A standardized extract of datura flower would be safer to use because the dosage of atropine and scopolamine could be precisely calculated, and the natural variation in the flower itself would be evened out by standardization.

Both standardized extracts and full–spectrum extracts have an important place in herbal medicine, but standardized extracts are somewhat uncommon in clinical Chinese medicine because there are relatively few herbs that are used based solely upon the pharmacology of their individual constituents. In many situations, the pharmacology and mechanisms of herbal compounds are poorly understood and it is thought that many variables beyond the known active constituents are involved in their activity. Thus the complex nature of full–spectrum extracts is preferred, and consumers tend to seek suppliers that have good surrounding quality control to ensure potency and efficacy despite the fact that the products are not standardized around specific compounds. That said, standardized extracts are of potential value for herbs that are highly variable in potency and possess well–characterized pharmacologic effects that can be traced to the activity of particular constituents that the plant contains.

3. Concentration Ratio

Concentration ratios are commonly used to measure potency in extract products. The concentration ratio is essentially a ratio that expresses the relationship between the raw herbs and the finished product. For example, if five kilograms of raw herbs are decocted and one kilogram of extract is obtained, this is called a 5:1 concentration (sometimes this would be called a 20% yield). This is often referred to as a Source:Product (S:P) ratio, because it is measuring the relationship between the raw materials and the finished product.

Concentration ratios can be confusing because there is no single standard across the industry. In Chinese medicine, we typically use full–spectrum water extracts and we express the concentration ratio as a relationship between the weights of the crude dried medicinals relative to the weight of the finished product. It is important to note that the concentration ratio should factor in the weight of any inactive excipients added to make the final product, but unfortunately this is not always the case. Generally speaking, if a granule product is said to have a concentration ratio of 9:1, we can assume that one gram of the granule powder is equivalent to nine grams of the raw herb.

Beyond the Chinese medicine industry, we see that some standardized extracts occasionally express concentration ratios based on isolated constituents. This is common for products such as gingko biloba leaves, which are often concentrated based on their active constituents for use in Western herbal medicine. Such products may list a concentration ratio of 50:1, which means that it would take 50 grams of the crude leaves to contain the constituents found in one gram of the finished product. This stands in contradistinction to the method used for full–spectrum extracts, such as those commonly used in Chinese medicine. In Chinese medicine, the concentration ratio typically refers to the amount of raw material relative to the finished product rather than focusing on the quantity of specific chemical constituents.

4. Marker Compounds

Marker compounds refer to chemical constituents within a medicinal that can be used to verify its potency or identity. For some medicinals, the marker compounds could be described as active ingredients. In other substances, the marker compounds of interest are chemicals that confirm the correct botanical identity of the starting material. There is not consensus on the correct marker compounds for all traditional medicinals, because some medicinals have unknown active constituents and others have multiple active constituents. In some situations, experts disagree about which group of constituents is responsible for the therapeutic effects of a given substance, so there is a lack of consensus when it comes to determining which constituents are the correct marker compounds for such items.

Items that have clear active ingredients often use these constituents as their marker compounds. This tends to give a reasonable method of assessing both potency and identity, but it is not a perfect system for definitively assessing quality. For example, the herb Ma Huang (Ephedrae

Herba) contains the active constituents ephedrine and pseudoephedrine, and these two constituents (or total ephedrine alkaloids) can be assessed to gauge its potency and identity. Different species of ephedra contain different quantities of the various ephedrine alkaloids, so assessing these therapeutic markers can tell us a lot about the source material and its strength. However, ephedra also contains volatile oils that may contribute to its medicinal effects, so looking at the ephedrine alkaloids alone provides an incomplete picture that cannot fully assess all aspects of product quality.

Similarly, the constituent berberine is thought to be a major active ingredient in Huang Lian (Coptidis Rhizoma), and the berberine content is often assessed when evaluating raw materials and finished products made from Huang Lian. However, berberine is not exclusive to Huang Lian, and can also be found in other herbs such as Huang Bai (Phellodendri Cortex). Thus, berberine can be used to generally assess the potency of Huang Lian, but it is not conclusive to verify the botanical identity of Huang Lian. Furthermore, berberine is also a constituent of the valuable Western herb goldenseal, and berberine content has in the past been used as a way of disguising adulteration in goldenseal products.

In some situations, our understanding of which marker compounds are the most important is incomplete or subject to revision. For example, the medicinal Dan Shen (Salviae Miltiorrhizae Radix) is often assessed based on a constituent called tanshinone IIA. However, Dan Shen has more than one active constituent and in recent years more and more attention has been given to its salvianolic acid content. In such cases, our understanding of which marker chemical is the most important to assess is constantly evolving, and analysis of multiple compounds may well be necessary to assess quality.

Items that have common problems with adulteration tend to use marker compounds as a means of assessing the botanical identity of the product. For example, the safe herb Han Fang Ji (Stephaniae Tetrandrae Radix) must be distinguished from the toxic substitute Guang Fang Ji (Aristolochiae Fangchi Radix). The two have a similar appearance and require chemical testing to definitively rule out adulteration by the toxic herb Guang Fang Ji. Han Fang Ji has a specific marker compound called tetrandrine that can be used to verify its identity, and Guang

Fang Ji has a marker compound called aristolochic acid that Han Fang Ji lacks. Thus, testing on Fang Ji products must verify that tetrandrine is present and aristolochic acid is absent. In this situation, tetrandrine happens to also be a compound with therapeutic activity, but the main purpose of the constituent testing for Fang Ji is focused on confirming botanical identity rather than measuring potency.

Finally, some products have unknown marker compounds. In the field of Chinese medicine, hundreds of plant, mineral, and animal products are used, and not all of these products have been studied in depth in terms of their chemistry and pharmacology. Multiple substances are typically used together and each medicinal is used in a variety of ways based on the unique paradigm of Chinese medicine, so it is difficult to know which chemicals are the active constituents for many items.

Pharmacologic studies of isolated constituents are often unable to capture the complexity of the polypharmacy approach and whole–plant preparations that characterize Chinese medicine, and the differences between Chinese medical theory and biomedicine further complicates a simple scientific explanation. For example, we can measure an herbal constituent's diuretic effect, but we have no method of evaluating its ability to calm liver yang. If the Chinese medical use of the substance focuses on calming liver yang, it is very hard to identify which constituent is responsible for that effect and it is likely that multiple constituents are involved. In some cases, the "active ingredient" may be formed from the interaction of two herbs together or may be due to a metabolite produced by the body rather than a natural constituent of the herb itself. These variables complicate the picture and make it challenging to identify the active constituents in Chinese herbs.

5. Jin Gao Fen (浸膏粉)

Jin gao fen is the Chinese name for a pure extract without any excipients. It is a powder made by evaporating the liquid of an extract. This is the strongest and purest form of an extract since it lacks excipients, but it tends to clump together once it is exposed to air. *Jin gao fen* can be packaged in single–dose foil packs or gelatin capsules, but it is rarely packaged loose in 100 gram bottles because it tends to clump rapidly. Most finished products contain excipients that help the product achieve its final consistency (such as loose granules or tablets). Pure *jin gao fen* extract is used in manufacturing, and excipients are added to it to make a variety of finished products.

6. Spray Drying

Spray drying is a term that is commonly used to describe the drying process when granules are manufactured. Spray drying uses a tall container of forced warm air to turn a viscous semiliquid extract into a dry powder. The semiliquid extract is sprayed into chamber and is dried by the forced air as it falls. This creates a dry extract powder that then is sieved to achieve a uniform consistency.

7. GMP

GMP stands for Good Manufacturing Practices. Different countries have slightly different GMP standards, and GMP standards vary from one industry to the next. In terms of granules, GMP laws generally require botanical identity testing, lot tracing, and many other details related to quality control and product tracking. The term cGMP refers to "current Good Manufacturing Practices" and cGMP is the term that is associated with U.S. FDA laws regarding GMP for dietary supplements (including granules).

8. Excipient

Excipients are materials that help a finished product achieve the correct consistency (such as a tablet, granule, tea pill, etc). Excipients in granules perform several important roles. Most importantly, excipients help the extract powder achieve a uniform consistency and prevent the powder from clumping together. The principle excipients used for granules include starch, dextrin, lactose, soluble dietary fiber, and cane sugar (usually only one of the above is used in any given product).

9. Ke Li (颗粒)

Ke li is the Chinese term for granule products that have a large particle size. Such products tend to be coarser than fine powders, and are particularly common in mainland China.

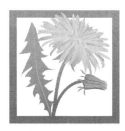

Commonly Used Formulas and Single Medicinals for Selected Conditions

Cough

1. Wind–cold cough

Formulas:

Ma Huang Tang (麻黄汤 Ephedra Decoction)

Xiao Qing Long Tang (小青龙汤 Minor Green–Blue Dragon Decoction)

Zhi Sou San (止嗽散 Cough–Stopping Powder)

San Ao Tang (三拗汤 Rough and Ready Three Decoction)

Single Medicinals:

Ma Huang (麻黄 Ephedra, Ephedrae Herba)

Zi Su Ye (紫苏叶 Perilla leaf, Perillae Folium)

Bai Qian (白前 Willowleaf swallowwort, Cynanchi Stauntonii Rhizoma)

Sheng Jiang (生姜 Fresh ginger, Zingiberis Rhizoma Recens)

Xing Ren (杏仁 Apricot kernel, Armeniacae Semen)

2. Wind–heat cough

Formulas:

Yin Qiao San (银翘散 Lonicera and Forsythia Powder)

Sang Ju Yin (桑菊饮 Mulberry Leaf and Chrysanthemum Beverage)

Ma Xing Shi Gan Tang (麻杏石甘汤 Ephedra, Apricot Kernel, Gypsum, and Licorice Decoction)

Single Medicinals:

Ju Hua (菊花 Chrysanthemum, Chrysanthemi Flos)

Sang Ye (桑叶 Mulberry leaf, Mori Folium)

Jie Geng (桔梗 Platycodon, Platycodonis Radix)

Niu Bang Zi (牛蒡子 Arctium, Arctii Fructus)

Lu Gen (芦根 Phragmites, Phragmitis Rhizoma)

Qian Hu (前胡 Peucedanum, Peucedani Radix)

3. Dryness–heat cough

Formulas:

Xing Su San (杏苏散 Apricot Kernel and Perilla Powder)

Qing Zao Jiu Fei Tang (清燥救肺汤 Dryness–Clearing Lung–Rescuing Decoction)

Bai He Gu Jin Tang (百合固金汤 Lily Bulb Metal–Securing Decoction)

Bei Mu Gua Lou San (贝母栝蒌散 Fritillaria and Trichosanthes Powder)

Sang Xing Tang (桑杏汤 Mulberry Leaf and Apricot Kernel Decoction)

Single Medicinals:

Zhi Mu (知母 Anemarrhena, Anemarrhenae Rhizoma)

Chuan Bei Mu (川贝母 Sichuan fritillaria, Fritillariae Cirrhosae Bulbus)

Sang Ye (桑叶 Mulberry leaf, Mori Folium)

Bai Bu (百部 Stemona, Stemonae Radix)

Fei Zi (榧子 Torreya, Torreyae Semen)

Zi Wan (紫菀 Aster, Asteris Radix)

Kuan Dong Hua (款冬花 Coltsfoot, Farfarae Flos)

Gan Cao (甘草 Licorice, Glycyrrhizae Radix)

4. Cold phlegm cough

Formulas:

Er Chen Tang (二陈汤 Two Matured Ingredients Decoction)

San Zi Yang Qin Tang (三子养亲汤 Three–Seed Filial Devotion Decoction)

Ling Gan Wu Wei Jiang Xin Tang (苓甘五味姜辛汤 Poria, Licorice, Schisandra, Ginger, and Asarum Decoction)

Xiao Qing Long Tang (小青龙汤 Minor Green–Blue Dragon Decoction)

Single Medicinals:

Tian Nan Xing (天南星 Arisaema, Arisaematis Rhizoma)

Bai Jie Zi (白芥子 White mustard, Sinapis Albae Semen)

Lai Fu Zi (莱菔子 Radish seed, Raphani Semen)

Xuan Fu Hua (旋覆花 Inula flower, Inulae Flos)

Zao Jia (皂荚 Gleditsia, Gleditsiae Fructus)

Bai Qian (白前 Willowleaf swallowwort, Cynanchi Stauntonii Rhizoma)

Gan Jiang (干姜 Dried ginger, Zingiberis Rhizoma)

Yuan Hua (芫花 Genkwa, Genkwa Flos)

5. Damp phlegm cough

Formulas:

Er Chen Tang (二陈汤 Two Matured Ingredients Decoction)

San Zi Yang Qin Tang (三子养亲汤 Three–Seed Filial Devotion Decoction)

Single Medicinals:

Tian Nan Xing (天南星 Arisaema, Arisaematis Rhizoma)

Ban Xia (半夏 Pinellia, Pinelliae Rhizoma)

Chen Pi (陈皮 Tangerine peel, Citri Reticulatae Pericarpium)

Fo Shou (佛手 Buddha's hand, Sacrodactylis Fructus)

Zao Jia (皂荚 Gleditsia, Gleditsiae Fructus)

Lai Fu Zi (莱菔子 Radish seed, Raphani Semen)

Yuan Hua (芫花 Genkwa, Genkwa Flos)

Zi Su Ye (紫苏叶 Perilla leaf, Perillae Folium)

6. Heat phlegm cough

Formulas:

Qing Jin Hua Tan Tang (清金化痰汤 Metal–Clearing Phlegm–Transforming Decoction)

Qing Qi Hua Tan Wan (清气化痰丸 Qi–Clearing Phlegm–Transforming Pill)

Xiao Xian Xiong Tang (小陷胸汤 Minor Chest Bind Decoction)

Gun Tan Wan (滚痰丸 Phlegm–Rolling Pill)

Single Medicinals:

Gua Lou (栝楼 Trichosanthes, Trichosanthis Fructus)

Bei Mu (贝母 Fritillaria, Fritillariae Bulbus)

Qian Hu (前胡 Peucedanum, Peucedani Radix)

Zhu Ru (竹茹 bamboo shavings, Bumbusae Caulis in Taenia)

Zhu Li (竹沥 Bamboo sap, Bambusae Succus)

Meng Shi (礞石 Chlorite/mica, Chloriti seu Micae Lapis)

Pang Da Hai (胖大海 Sterculia, Sterculiae Lychnophorae Semen)

Sang Bai Pi (桑白皮 Mulberry root bark, Mori Cortex)

Di Gu Pi (地骨皮 Lycium root bark, Lycii Cortex)

Zhi Mu (知母 Anemarrhena, Anemarrhenae Rhizoma)

Dan Xing (胆星 Bile arisaema, Arisaema cum Bile)

Tian Zhu Huang (天竹黄 Bamboo sugar, Bambusae Concretio Silicea)

Hu Zhang (虎杖 Bushy knotweed, Polygoni Cuspidati Rhizoma)

Che Qian Zi (车前子 Plantago seed, Plantaginis Semen)

Shi Wei (石韦 Pyrrosia, Pyrrosiae Folium)

Ce Bai Ye (侧柏叶 Arborvitae leaf, Platycladi Cacumen)

Chuan Xin Lian (穿心莲 Andrographis, Andrographis Herba)

She Gan (射干 Belamcanda, Belamcandae Rhizoma)

Shan Dou Gen (山豆根 Vietnamese sophora, Sophorae Tonkinensi Radix)

Qing Dai (青黛 Indigo, Indigo Naturalis)

Peng Sha (硼砂 Borax, Borax)

7. Qi vacuity cough

Formulas:

Ren Shen Ge Jie San (人参蛤蚧散 Ginseng and Gecko Powder)

Sheng Mai San (生脉散 Pulse-Engendering Powder)

Shen Su Yin (参苏饮 Ginseng and Perilla Beverage)

Bai Du San (败毒散 Toxin-Vanquishing Powder)

Single Medicinals:

Ren Shen (人参 Ginseng, Ginseng Radix)

Xi Yang Shen (西洋参 American ginseng, Panacis Quinquefolii Radix)

·Dang Shen (党参 Codonopsis, Codonopsis Radix)

Tai Zi Shen (太子参 Pseudostellaria, Pseudostellariae Radix)

Huang Qi (黄芪 Astragalus, Astragali Radix)

Wu Wei Zi (五味子 Schisandra, Schisandrae Fructus)

Ge Jie (蛤蚧 Gecko, Gecko)

Shan Yao (山药 Dioscorea, Dioscoreae Rhizoma)

Yi Tang (饴糖 Malt sugar, Maltosum)

Hu Tao Ren (胡桃仁 Walnut, Juglandis Semen)

Feng Mi (蜂蜜 Honey, Mel)

Ying Su Ke (Qiao) (罂粟壳 Poppy husk, Papaveris Pericarpium)

He Zi (诃子 Chebule, Chebulae Fructus)

Wu Bei Zi (五倍子 Sumac gallnut, Galla Chinensis)

Wu Mei (乌梅 Mume, Mume Fructus)

8. Yin vacuity cough

Formulas:

Sha Shen Mai Dong Tang (沙参麦冬汤 Adenophora/glehnia and Ophiopogon Decoction)

Bai He Gu Jin Tang (百合固金汤 Lily Bulb Metal–Securing Decoction)

Qing Zao Jiu Fei Tang (清燥救肺汤 Dryness–Clearing Lung–Rescuing Decoction)

Sheng Mai San (生脉散 Pulse–Engendering Powder)

Liu Wei Di Huang Wan (六味地黄丸 Six–Ingredient Rehmannia Pill)

Zhi Bai Di Huang Wan (知柏地黄丸 Anemarrhena, Phellodendron, and Rehmannia Pill)

Bu Fei Tang (补肺汤 Lung–Supplementing Decoction)

Jiu Xian San (九仙散 Nine Immortals Powder)

Yu Zhu (玉竹 Solomon's seal, Polygonati Odorati Rhizoma)

Sha Shen (沙参 Adenophora/glehnia, Adenophorae seu Glehniae Radix)

Mai Men Dong (麦门冬 Ophiopogon, Ophiopogonis Radix)

Tian Men Dong (天门冬 Asparagus, Asparagi Radix)

Bai He (百合 Lily bulb, Lilii Bulbus)

Huang Jing (黄精 Polygonatum, Polygonati Rhizoma)

Bai Bu (百部 Stemona, Stemonae Radix)

Chuan Bei Mu (川贝母 Sichuan fritillaria, Fritillariae Cirrhosae Bulbus)

Zhi Mu (知母 Anemarrhena, Anemarrhenae Rhizoma)

Gou Qi Zi (枸杞子 Lycium, Lycii Fructus)

E Jiao (阿胶 Ass hide glue, Asini Corii Colla)

9. Lung heat cough

Formulas:

Sang Ju Yin (桑菊饮 Mulberry Leaf and Chrysanthemum Beverage)

Ma Xing Shi Gan Tang (麻杏石甘汤 Ephedra, Apricot Kernel, Gypsum, and Licorice Decoction)

Xie Bai San (泻白散 White–Draining Powder)

Qing Qi Hua Tan Wan (清气化痰丸 Qi–Clearing Phlegm–Transforming Pill)

Single Medicinals:

Shi Gao (石膏 Gypsum, Gypsum Fibrosum)

Huang Qin (黄芩 Scutellaria, Scutellariae Radix)

Lu Gen (芦根 Phragmites, Phragmitis Rhizoma)

Zhi Mu (知母 Anemarrhena, Anemarrhenae Rhizoma)

Tian Hua Fen (天花粉 Trichosanthes root, Trichosanthis Radix)

Chuan Xin Lian (穿心莲 Andrographis, Andrographis Herba)

Ma Bo (马勃 Puffball, Lasiosphaera seu Calvatia)

Yu Xing Cao (鱼腥草 Houttuynia, Houttuyniae Herba)

Di Gu Pi (地骨皮 Lycium root bark, Lycii Cortex)

Xia Ku Cao (夏枯草 Prunella, Prunellae Spica)

Che Qian Zi (车前子 Plantago seed, Plantaginis Semen)

Shi Wei (石韦 Pyrrosia, Pyrrosiae Folium)

Bai Mao Gen (白茅根 Imperata, Imperatae Rhizoma)

Hu Zhang (虎杖 Bushy knotweed, Polygoni Cuspidati Rhizoma)

Zhu Ru (竹茹 Bamboo shavings, Bumbusae Caulis in Taenia)

Er Cha (儿茶 Cutch, Catechu)

Panting

1. Cold panting

Formulas:

Ma Huang Tang (麻黄汤 Ephedra Decoction)

San Ao Tang (三拗汤 Rough and Ready Three Decoction)

Xiao Qing Long Tang (小青龙汤 Minor Green–Blue Dragon Decoction)

Ding Chuan Tang (定喘汤 Panting–Stabilizing Decoction)

Single Medicinals:

Ma Huang (麻黄 Ephedra, Ephedrae Herba)

Xing Ren (杏仁 Apricot kernel, Armeniacae Semen)

Zi Su Zi (紫苏子 Perilla fruit, Perillae Fructus)

Lai Fu Zi (莱菔子 Radish seed, Raphani Semen)

Bai Jie Zi (白芥子 White mustard, Sinapis Albae Semen)

Yang Jin Hua (洋金花 Datura flower, Daturae Flos)

Ci Shi (磁石 Loadstone, Magnetitum)

Gan Jiang (干姜 Dried ginger, Zingiberis Rhizoma)

Xi Xin (细辛 Asarum, Asari Herba)

2. Heat panting

Formulas:

Ma Xing Shi Gan Tang (麻杏石甘汤 Ephedra, Apricot Kernel, Gypsum, and Licorice Decoction)

Sang Bai Pi Tang (桑白皮汤 Mulberry Root Bark Decoction)

Single Medicinals:

Sang Bai Pi (桑白皮 Mulberry root bark, Mori Cortex)

Bai Guo (白果 Ginkgo, Ginkgo Semen)

Huang Qin (黄芩 Scutellaria, Scutellariae Radix)

Ting Li Zi (葶苈子 Lepidium/descurainiae, Lepidii/Descurainiae Semen)

Qian Hu (前胡 Peucedanum, Peucedani Radix)

Shi Wei (石韦 Pyrrosia, Pyrrosiae Folium)

Pi Pa Ye (枇杷叶 Loquat leaf, Eriobotryae Folium)

3. Phlegm turbidity panting

Formulas:

Er Chen Tang (二陈汤 Two Matured Ingredients Decoction)

San Zi Yang Qin Tang (三子养亲汤 Three-Seed Filial Devotion Decoction)

Gun Tan Wan (滚痰丸 Phlegm-Rolling Pill)

Single Medicinals:

Hou Po (厚朴 Official magnolia bark, Magnoliae Officinalis Cortex)

Bai Guo (白果 Ginkgo, Ginkgo Semen)

Xiong Huang (雄黄 Realgar, Realgar)

4. Lung vacuity panting

Formulas:

Yu Ping Feng San (玉屏风散 Jade Wind–Barrier Powder)

Ren Shen Ge Jie San (人参蛤蚧散 Ginseng and Gecko Powder)

Sheng Mai San (生脉散 Pulse–Engendering Powder)

Single Medicinals:

Ren Shen (人参 Ginseng, Ginseng Radix)

Dang Shen (党参 Codonopsis, Codonopsis Radix)

Shan Yao (山药 Dioscorea, Dioscoreae Rhizoma)

Mai Men Dong (麦门冬 Ophiopogon, Ophiopogonis Radix)

Wu Wei Zi (五味子 Schisandra, Schisandrae Fructus)

5. Kidney yang vacuity panting

Formulas:

Qi Wei Du Qi Wan (七味都气丸 Seven–Ingredient Metropolis Qi Pill)

Shen Qi Wan (肾气丸 Kidney Qi Pill)

Ren Shen Ge Jie San (人参蛤蚧散 Ginseng and Gecko Powder)

Single Medicinals:

Fu Zi (附子 Aconite, Aconiti Radix Lateralis Praeparata)

Bu Gu Zhi (补骨脂 Psoralea, Psoraleae Fructus)

Ge Jie (蛤蚧 Gecko, Gecko)

6. Lung–kidney vacuity panting

Formulas:

Ren Shen Ge Jie San (人参蛤蚧散 Ginseng and Gecko Powder)

Sheng Mai San (生脉散 Pulse–Engendering Powder)

Single Medicinals:

Dong Chong Xia Cao (冬虫夏草 Cordyceps, Cordyceps)

Hu Tao Ren (胡桃仁 Walnut, Juglandis Semen)

Ge Jie (蛤蚧 Gecko, Gecko)

Zi He Che (紫河车 Placenta, Hominis Placenta)

Ci Shi (磁石 Loadstone, Magnetitum)

Headache

1. Wind–cold headache

Formulas:

Chuan Xiong Cha Tiao San (川芎茶调散 Tea–Blended Chuanxiong Powder)

Ma Huang Xi Xin Fu Zi Tang (麻黄细辛附子汤 Ephedra, Asarum, and Aconite Decoction) with concurrent kidney yang vacuity

Single Medicinals:

Ma Huang (麻黄 Ephedra, Ephedrae Herba)

Gui Zhi (桂枝 Cinnamon twig, Cinnamomi Ramulus)

Zi Su Ye (紫苏叶 Perilla leaf, Perillae Folium)

Xiang Ru (香薷 Mosla, Moslae Herba)

Xin Yi (辛夷 Magnolia flower, Magnoliae Flos)

Cang Er Zi (苍耳子 Xanthium, Xanthii Fructus)

Fang Feng (防风 Saposhnikovia, Saposhnikoviae Radix)

Qiang Huo (羌活 Notopterygium, Notopterygii Rhizoma et Radix)

Jing Jie (荆芥 Schizonepeta, Schizonepetae Herba)

Bai Zhi (白芷 Dahurian angelica, Angelicae Dahuricae Radix)

Xi Xin (细辛 Asarum, Asari Herba)

Gao Ben (藁本 Chinese lovage, Ligustici Rhizoma)

Chuan Xiong (川芎 Chuanxiong, Chuanxiong Rhizoma)

2. Wind–heat headache

Formulas:

Ju Hua Cha Tiao San (菊花茶调散 Tea–Blended Chrysanthemum Powder)

Xiong Zhi Shi Gao Tang (芎芷石膏汤 Chuanxiong, Dahurian Angelica, and Gypsum Decoction)

Single Medicinals:

Sang Ye (桑叶 Mulberry leaf, Mori Folium)

Ju Hua (菊花 Chrysanthemum, Chrysanthemi Flos)

Bo He (薄荷 Mint, Menthae Herba)

Jing Jie (荆芥 Schizonepeta, Schizonepetae Herba)

Niu Bang Zi (牛蒡子 Arctium, Arctii Fructus)

Jiang Can (僵蚕 Silkworm, Bombyx Batryticatus)

Dan Dou Chi (淡豆豉 Fermented soybean, Sojae Semen Praeparatum)

Chan Tui (蝉蜕 Cicada molting, Cicadae Periostracum)

Mu Zei (木贼 Equisetum, Equiseti Hiemalis Herba)

Jin Yin Hua (金银花 Lonicera, Lonicerae Flos)

Lian Qiao (连翘 Forsythia, Forsythiae Fructus)

3. Wind–damp headache

Formulas:

Qiang Huo Sheng Shi Tang (羌活胜湿汤 Notopterygium Dampness–Overcoming Decoction)

Single Medicinals:

Qiang Huo (羌活 Notopterygium, Notopterygii Rhizoma et Radix)

Fang Feng (防风 Saposhnikovia, Saposhnikoviae Radix)

Bai Zhi (白芷 Dahurian angelica, Angelicae Dahuricae Radix)

Chuan Xiong (川芎 Chuanxiong, Chuanxiong Rhizoma)

Cang Er Zi (苍耳子 Xanthium, Xanthii Fructus)

Du Huo (独活 Pubescent angelica, Angelicae Pubescentis Radix)

Gao Ben (藁本 Chinese lovage, Ligustici Rhizoma)

4. Liver yang headache

Formulas:

Tian Ma Gou Teng Yin (天麻钩藤饮 Gastrodia and Uncaria Beverage)

Single Medicinals:

Tian Ma (天麻 Gastrodia, Gastrodiae Rhizoma)

Gou Teng (钩藤 Uncaria, Uncariae Ramulus cum Uncis)

Bai Ji Li (白蒺藜 Tribulus, Tribuli Fructus)

Zhen Zhu Mu (珍珠母 Mother-of-pearl, Concha Margaritifera)

Dai Zhe Shi (代赭石 Hematite, Haematitum)

Ci Shi (磁石 Loadstone, Magnetitum)

Ju Hua (菊花 Chrysanthemum, Chrysanthemi Flos)

Lu Dou Yi (绿豆衣 Mung bean seed-coat, Phaseoli Radiati Testa)

Ling Yang Jiao (羚羊角 Antelope horn, Saigae Tataricae Cornu)

Shi Jue Ming (石决明 Abalone shell, Haliotidis Concha)

Long Gu (龙骨 Dragon bone, Mastodi Ossis Fossilia)

Mu Li (牡蛎 Oyster shell, Ostreae Concha)

Huai Hua (槐花 Sophora flower, Sophorae Flos)

5. Liver fire headache

Formulas:

Long Dan Xie Gan Tang (龙胆泻肝汤 Gentian Liver-Draining Decoction)

Xie Qing Wan (泻青丸 Green-Blue-Draining Pill)

Single Medicinals:

Xia Ku Cao (夏枯草 Prunella, Prunellae Spica)

Long Dan (龙胆 Gentian, Gentianae Radix)

Ling Yang Jiao (羚羊角 Antelope horn, Saigae Tataricae Cornu)

Jue Ming Zi (决明子 Fetid cassia, Cassiae Semen)

Shi Jue Ming (石决明 Abalone shell, Haliotidis Concha)

Jiang Can (僵蚕 Silkworm, Bombyx Batryticatus)

Ju Hua (菊花 Chrysanthemum, Chrysanthemi Flos)

6. Qi vacuity headache

Formulas:

Bu Zhong Yi Qi Tang (补中益气汤 Center–Supplementing Qi–Boosting Decoction)

Si Jun Zi Tang (四君子汤 Four Gentlemen Decoction)

Single Medicinals:

Ren Shen (人参 Ginseng, Ginseng Radix)

Dang Shen (党参 Codonopsis, Codonopsis Radix)

Huang Qi (黄芪 Astragalus, Astragali Radix)

Sheng Ma (升麻 Cimicifuga, Cimicifugae Rhizoma)

Ge Gen (葛根 Pueraria, Puerariae Radix)

Chai Hu (柴胡 Bupleurum, Bupleuri Radix)

Xi Yang Shen (西洋参 American ginseng, Panacis Quinquefolii Radix)

Tai Zi Shen (太子参 Pseudostellaria, Pseudostellariae Radix)

7. Kidney vacuity headache

Formulas:

Da Bu Yuan Jian (大补元煎 Major Origin–Supplementing Brew) – Yin vacuity

You Gui Wan (右归丸 Right–Restoring Pill) – Yang vacuity

Ma Huang Xi Xin Fu Zi Tang (麻黄细辛附子汤 Ephedra, Asarum, and Aconite Decoction) – Yang vacuity with wind–cold

Single Medicinals:

Shan Zhu Yu (山茱萸 Cornus, Corni Fructus)

He Shou Wu (何首乌 Flowery knotweed, Polygoni Multiflori Radix)

Gou Qi Zi (枸杞子 Lycium, Lycii Fructus)

Shu Di Huang (熟地黄 Cooked rehmannia, Rehmanniae Radix Praeparata)

8. Blood vacuity headache

Formulas:

Si Wu Tang (四物汤 Four Agents Decoction)

Gui Pi Tang (归脾汤 Spleen–Returning Decoction)

Single Medicinals:

Dang Gui (当归 Chinese angelica, Angelicae Sinensis Radix)

Shu Di Huang (熟地黄 Cooked rehmannia, Rehmanniae Radix Praeparata)

Bai Shao Yao (白芍药 White peony, Paeoniae Radix Alba)

Sang Shen (桑椹 Mulberry, Mori Fructus)

Gou Qi Zi (枸杞子 Lycium, Lycii Fructus)

He Shou Wu (何首乌 Flowery knotweed, Polygoni Multiflori Radix)

Lu Dou Yi (绿豆衣 Mung bean seed–coat, Phaseoli Radiati Testa)

Ju Hua (菊花 Chrysanthemum, Chrysanthemi Flos)

Man Jing Zi (蔓荆子 Vitex, Viticis Fructus)

9. Blood stasis headache

Formulas:

Tong Qiao Huo Xue Tang (通窍活血汤 Orifice–Freeing Blood–Quickening Decoction)

Single Medicinals:

Chuan Xiong (川芎 Chuanxiong, Chuanxiong Rhizoma)

Niu Xi (牛膝 Achyranthes, Achyranthis Bidentatae Radix)

She Xiang (麝香 Musk, Moschus)

Yu Jin (郁金 Curcuma, Curcumae Radix)

Bai Zhi (白芷 Dahurian angelica, Angelicae Dahuricae Radix)

Quan Xie (全蝎 Scorpion, Scorpio)

Wu Gong (蜈蚣 Centipede, Scolopendra)

Zhe Chong (蟅虫 Ground beetle, Eupolyphaga seu Steleophaga)

Yan Hu Suo (延胡索 Corydalis, Corydalis Rhizoma)

10. Phlegm turbidity headache

Formulas:

Ban Xia Bai Zhu Tian Ma Tang (半夏白朮天麻汤 Pinellia, White Atractylodes, and Gastrodia Decoction)

Single Medicinals:

Bai Fu Zi (白附子 Typhonium, Typhonii Rhizoma)

Bai Zhu (白朮 White atractylodes, Atractylodis Macrocephalae Rhizoma)

Hou Po (厚朴 Officinal magnolia bark, Magnoliae Officinalis Cortex)

Bai Ji Li (白蒺藜 Tribulus, Tribuli Fructus)

Man Jing Zi (蔓荆子 Vitex, Viticis Fructus)

Ban Xia (半夏 Pinellia, Pinelliae Rhizoma)

Dizziness

1. Liver yang dizziness

Formulas:

Tian Ma Gou Teng Yin (天麻钩藤饮 Gastrodia and Uncaria Beverage)

Da Ding Feng Zhu (大定风珠 Major Wind–Stabilizing Pill)

Single Medicinals:

Tian Ma (天麻 Gastrodia, Gastrodiae Rhizoma)

Gou Teng (钩藤 Uncaria, Uncariae Ramulus cum Uncis)

Shi Jue Ming (石决明 Abalone shell, Haliotidis Concha)

Jue Ming Zi (决明子 Fetid cassia, Cassiae Semen)

Xia Ku Cao (夏枯草 Prunella, Prunellae Spica)

Long Gu (龙骨 dragon bone, Mastodi Ossis Fossilia)

Mu Li (牡蛎 Oyster shell, Ostreae Concha)

Ci Shi (磁石 Loadstone, Magnetitum)

Dai Zhe Shi (代赭石 Hematite, Haematitum)

Zhen Zhu Mu (珍珠母 Mother-of-pearl, Concha Margaritifera)

Gui Ban (龟板 Tortoise shell, Testudinis Carapax et Plastrum)

Bai Shao Yao (白芍药 White peony, Paeoniae Radix Alba)

Du Zhong (杜仲 Eucommia, Eucommiae Cortex)

Ju Hua (菊花 Chrysanthemum, Chrysanthemi Flos)

Bai Ji Li (白蒺藜 Tribulus, Tribuli Fructus)

Ling Yang Jiao (羚羊角 Antelope horn, Saigae Tataricae Cornu)

Lu Dou Yi (绿豆衣 Mung bean seed-coat, Phaseoli Radiati Testa)

2. Liver fire dizziness

Formulas:

Long Dan Xie Gan Tang (龙胆泻肝汤 Gentian Liver-Draining Decoction)

Dang Gui Long Hui Wan (当归龙荟丸 Chinese Angelica, Gentian, and Aloe Pill)

Single Medicinals:

Xia Ku Cao (夏枯草 Prunella, Prunellae Spica)

Long Dan (龙胆 Gentian, Gentianae Radix)

Ling Yang Jiao (羚羊角 Antelope horn, Saigae Tataricae Cornu)

Ju Hua (菊花 Chrysanthemum, Chrysanthemi Flos)

Lu Hui (芦荟 Aloe, Aloe)

Gou Teng (钩藤 Uncaria, Uncariae Ramulus cum Uncis)

Huai Hua (槐花 Sophora flower, Sophorae Flos)

3. Liver wind dizziness

Formulas:

Zhen Gan Xi Feng Tang (镇肝熄风汤 Liver–Settling Wind–Extinguishing Decoction)

Tian Ma Gou Teng Yin (天麻钩藤饮 Gastrodia and Uncaria Beverage)

E Jiao Ji Zi Huang Tang (阿胶鸡子黄汤 Ass Hide Glue and Egg Yolk Decoction)

Da Ding Feng Zhu (大定风珠 Major Wind–Stabilizing Pill)

Single Medicinals:

Ling Yang Jiao (羚羊角 Antelope horn, Saigae Tataricae Cornu)

Gou Teng (钩藤 Uncaria, Uncariae Ramulus cum Uncis)

Tian Ma (天麻 Gastrodia, Gastrodiae Rhizoma)

Ju Hua (菊花 Chrysanthemum, Chrysanthemi Flos)

4. Blood vacuity dizziness

Formulas:

Si Wu Tang (四物汤 Four Agents Decoction)

Gui Pi Tang (归脾汤 Spleen–Returning Decoction)

Single Medicinals:

Dang Gui (当归 Chinese angelica, Angelicae Sinensis Radix)

Shu Di Huang (熟地黄 Cooked rehmannia, Rehmanniae Radix Praeparata)

Bai Shao Yao (白芍药 White peony, Paeoniae Radix Alba)

E Jiao (阿胶 Ass hide glue, Asini Corii Colla)

Long Yan Rou (龙眼肉 Longan flesh, Longan Arillus)

He Shou Wu (何首乌 Flowery knotweed, Polygoni Multiflori Radix)

Sang Shen (桑椹 Mulberry, Mori Fructus)

Lu Dou Yi (绿豆衣 Mung bean seed–coat, Phaseoli Radiati Testa)

Zi He Che (紫河车 Placenta, Hominis Placenta)

5. Qi vacuity dizziness

Formulas:

Bu Zhong Yi Qi Tang (补中益气汤 Center–Supplementing Qi–Boosting Decoction)

Gui Pi Tang (归脾汤 Spleen–Returning Decoction)

Single Medicinals:

Ren Shen (人参 Ginseng, Ginseng Radix)

Dang Shen (党参 Codonopsis, Codonopsis Radix)

Huang Qi (黄芪 Astragalus, Astragali Radix)

Xi Yang Shen (西洋参 American ginseng, Panacis Quinquefolii Radix)

Tai Zi Shen (太子参 Pseudostellaria, Pseudostellariae Radix)

6. Yin vacuity dizziness

Formulas:

Qi Ju Di Huang Wan (杞菊地黄丸 Lycium Berry, Chrysanthemum, and Rehmannia Pill)

Single Medicinals:

Shu Di Huang (熟地黄 Cooked rehmannia, Rehmanniae Radix Praeparata)

Shan Zhu Yu (山茱萸 Cornus, Corni Fructus)

Shan Yao (山药 Dioscorea, Dioscoreae Rhizoma)

Huang Jing (黄精 Polygonatum, Polygonati Rhizoma)

Gou Qi Zi (枸杞子 Lycium, Lycii Fructus)

Sang Shen (桑椹 Mulberry, Mori Fructus)

Mo Han Lian (墨旱莲 Eclipta, Ecliptae Herba)

Nu Zhen Zi (女贞子 Ligustrum, Ligustri Lucidi Fructus)

Hei Zhi Ma (黑脂麻 Black sesame, Sesami Semen Nigrum)

Zi He Che (紫河车 Placenta, Hominis Placenta)

He Shou Wu (何首乌 Flowery knotweed, Polygoni Multiflori Radix)

7. Yang vacuity dizziness

Formulas:

You Gui Wan (右归丸 Right–Restoring [Life Gate] Pill)

Single Medicinals:

Lu Rong (鹿茸 Velvet deerhorn, Cervi Cornu Pantotrichum)

Zi He Che (紫河车 Placenta, Hominis Placenta)

Sha Yuan Zi (沙苑子 Complanate astragalus seed, Astragali Complanati Semen)

Shan Zhu Yu (山茱萸 Cornus, Corni Fructus)

Tu Si Zi (菟丝子 Cuscuta, Cuscutae Semen)

8. Phlegm turbidity dizziness

Formulas:

Ban Xia Bai Zhu Tian Ma Tang (半夏白术天麻汤 Pinellia, White Atractylodes, and Gastrodia Decoction)

Single Medicinals:

Tian Nan Xing (天南星 Arisaema, Arisaematis Rhizoma)

Ban Xia (半夏 Pinellia, Pinelliae Rhizoma)

Bai Zhu (白术 White atractylodes, Atractylodis Macrocephalae Rhizoma)

Ze Xie (泽泻 Alisma, Alismatis Rhizoma)

Fu Ling (茯苓 Poria, Poria)

Zhu Ru (竹茹 Bamboo shavings, Bumbusae Caulis in Taenia)

Eye Diseases

1. Wind–heat of the eye

Formulas:

Sang Xing Tang (桑杏汤 Mulberry Leaf and Apricot Kernel Decoction)

Yin Qiao San (银翘散 Lonicera and Forsythia Powder)

Single Medicinals:

Sang Ye (桑叶 Mulberry leaf, Mori Folium)

Bo He (薄荷 Mint, Menthae Herba)

Ju Hua (菊花 Chrysanthemum, Chrysanthemi Flos)

Mu Zei (木贼 Equisetum, Equiseti Hiemalis Herba)

Chi Shao Yao (赤芍药 Red peony, Paeoniae Radix Rubra)

Bai Ji Li (白蒺藜 Tribulus, Tribuli Fructus)

Jiang Can (僵蚕 Silkworm, Bombyx Batryticatus)

Chan Tui (蝉蜕 Cicada molting, Cicadae Periostracum)

Jue Ming Zi (决明子 Fetid cassia, Cassiae Semen)

Man Jing Zi (蔓荆子 Vitex, Viticis Fructus)

2. Liver heat of the eye

Formulas:

Long Dan Xie Gan Tang (龙胆泻肝汤 Gentian Liver–Draining Decoction)

Dang Gui Long Hui Wan (当归龙荟丸 Chinese Angelica, Gentian, and Aloe Pill)

Single Medicinals:

Ju Hua (菊花 Chrysanthemum, Chrysanthemi Flos)

Sang Ye (桑叶 Mulberry leaf, Mori Folium)

Xia Ku Cao (夏枯草 Prunella, Prunellae Spica)

Chi Shao Yao (赤芍药 Red peony, Paeoniae Radix Rubra)

Zi Hua Di Ding (紫花地丁 Violet, Violae Herba)

Qin Pi (秦皮 Ash, Fraxini Cortex)

Jue Ming Zi (决明子 Fetid cassia, Cassiae Semen)

Shi Jue Ming (石决明 Abalone shell, Haliotidis Concha)

Ling Yang Jiao (羚羊角 Antelope horn, Saigae Tataricae Cornu)

Zhen Zhu Mu (珍珠母 Mother–of–pearl, Concha Margaritifera)

Zhen Zhu (珍珠 Pearl, Margarita)

Che Qian Zi (车前子 Plantago seed, Plantaginis Semen)

Chong Wei Zi (茺蔚子 Leonurus fruit, Leonuri Fructus)

Da Huang (大黄 Rhubarb, Rhei Radix et Rhizoma)

Mang Xiao (芒硝 Mirabilite, Natrii Sulfas)

Jiang Can (僵蚕 Silkworm, Bombyx Batryticatus)

3. Liver vacuity clouded vision

Formulas:

Yi Guan Jian (一贯煎 All–the–Way–Through Brew)

Si Wu Tang (四物汤 Four Agents Decoction)

Qi Ju Di Huang Wan (杞菊地黄丸 Lycium Berry, Chrysanthemum, and Rehmannia Pill)

Ming Mu Di Huang Wan (明目地黄丸 Eye Brightener Rehmannia Pill)

Single Medicinals:

Sha Yuan Zi (沙苑子 Complanate astragalus seed, Astragali Complanati Semen)

Tu Si Zi (菟丝子 Cuscuta, Cuscutae Semen)

Shi Hu (石斛 Dendrobium, Dendrobii Herba)

Gou Qi Zi (枸杞子 Lycium, Lycii Fructus)

Sang Shen (桑椹 Mulberry, Mori Fructus)

Nu Zhen Zi (女贞子 Ligustrum, Ligustri Lucidi Fructus)

Hei Zhi Ma (黑脂麻 Black sesame, Sesami Semen Nigrum)

Toothache

1. Stomach fire (gum swelling and pain)

Formulas:

Qing Wei San (清胃散 Stomach–Clearing Powder)

Yu Nu Jian (玉女煎 Jade Lady Brew)

Single Medicinals:

Shi Gao (石膏 Gypsum, Gypsum Fibrosum)

Sheng Ma (升麻 Cimicifuga, Cimicifugae Rhizoma)

Huang Lian (黄连 Coptis, Coptidis Rhizoma)

Da Huang (大黄 Rhubarb, Rhei Radix et Rhizoma)

Zhu Ye (竹叶 Bamboo leaf, Lophatheri Folium)

Bai Zhi (白芷 Dahurian angelica, Angelicae Dahuricae Radix)

2. Toothache from kidney vacuity (gum pain)

Formulas:

Zhi Bai Di Huang Wan (知柏地黄丸 Anemarrhena, Phellodendron, and Rehmannia Pill)

You Gui Wan (右归丸 Right–Restoring Pill)

Zuo Gui Wan (左归丸 Left–Restoring Pill)

Single Medicinals:

Gu Sui Bu (骨碎补 Drynaria, Drynariae Rhizoma)

Xi Xin (细辛 Asarum, Asari Herba)

Gou Ji (狗脊 Cibotium, Cibotii Rhizoma)

Niu Xi (牛膝 Achyranthes, Achyranthis Bidentatae Radix)

3. Toothache from wind–cold

Formulas:

Ma Huang Xi Xin Fu Zi Tang (麻黄细辛附子汤 Ephedra, Asarum, and Aconite Decoction)

Single Medicinals:

Bai Zhi (白芷 Dahurian angelica, Angelicae Dahuricae Radix)

Gao Ben (藁本 Chinese lovage, Ligustici Rhizoma)

Xi Xin (细辛 Asarum, Asari Herba)

Sore Throat

1. Wind–heat sore throat

Formulas:

Yin Qiao San (银翘散 Lonicera and Forsythia Powder)

Sang Ju Yin (桑菊饮 Mulberry Leaf and Chrysanthemum Beverage)

Single Medicinals:

Bo He (薄荷 Mint, Menthae Herba)

Niu Bang Zi (牛蒡子 Arctium, Arctii Fructus)

Sang Ye (桑叶 Mulberry leaf, Mori Folium)

Jiang Can (僵蚕 Silkworm, Bombyx Batryticatus)

Sheng Ma (升麻 Cimicifuga, Cimicifugae Rhizoma)

2. Vacuity fire sore throat

Formulas:

Zhi Bai Di Huang Wan (知柏地黄丸 Anemarrhena, Phellodendron, and Rehmannia Pill)

Zeng Ye Tang (增液汤 Humor–Increasing Decoction)

Single Medicinals:

Xuan Shen (玄参 Scrophularia, Scrophulariae Radix)

Sheng Di Huang (生地黄 Dried/fresh rehmannia, Rehmanniae Radix Exsiccata seu Recens)

Zhi Mu (知母 Anemarrhena, Anemarrhenae Rhizoma)

Huang Bai (黄柏 Phellodendron, Phellodendri Cortex)

3. Repletion fire sore throat

Formulas:

Bai Hu Tang (白虎汤 White Tiger Decoction)

Zhu Ye Shi Gao Tang (竹叶石膏汤 Lophatherum and Gypsum Decoction)

Single Medicinals:

Shan Dou Gen (山豆根 Vietnamese sophora, Sophorae Tonkinensis Radix)

Ma Bo (马勃 Puffball, Lasiosphaera seu Calvatia)

She Gan (射干 Belamcanda, Belamcandae Rhizoma)

Niu Bang Zi (牛蒡子 Arctium, Arctii Fructus)

Jing Jie (荆芥 Schizonepeta, Schizonepetae Herba)

Jie Geng (桔梗 Platycodon, Platycodonis Radix)

Lian Qiao (连翘 Forsythia, Forsythiae Fructus)

Gan Cao (甘草 Licorice, Glycyrrhizae Radix)

4. Heat toxin sore throat

Formulas:

Pu Ji Xiao Du Yin (普济消毒饮 Universal Salvation Toxin–Dispersing Beverage)

Liang Ge San (凉膈散 Diaphragm–Cooling Powder)

Wu Wei Xiao Du Yin (五味消毒饮 Five–Ingredient Toxin–Dispersing Beverage)

Yin Qiao San (银翘散 Lonicera and Forsythia Powder)

Single Medicinals:

Ban Lan Gen (板蓝根 Isatis root, Isatidis Radix)

Da Qing Ye (大青叶 Isatis leaf, Isatidis Folium)

Jin Yin Hua (金银花 Lonicera, Lonicerae Flos)

Lian Qiao (连翘 Forsythia, Forsythiae Fructus)

Chuan Xin Lian (穿心莲 Andrographis, Andrographis Herba)

Niu Huang (牛黄 Bovine bezoar, Bovis Calculus)

Bai Hua She She Cao (白花蛇舌草 Oldenlandia, Oldenlandiae Diffusae Herba)

Xia Ku Cao (夏枯草 Prunella, Prunellae Spica)

Zhu Sha (朱砂 Cinnabar, Cinnabaris)

Da Huang (大黄 Rhubarb, Rhei Radix et Rhizoma)

Mang Xiao (芒硝 Mirabilite, Natrii Sulfas)

Deng Xin Cao (灯心草 Juncus, Junci Medulla)

Deep–Source Nasal Congestion

Formulas:

Cang Er Zi San (苍耳子散 Xanthium Powder)

Xin Yi San (辛夷散 Officinal Magnolia Flower Powder)

Xin Yi Qing Fei Tang (辛夷清肺汤 Officinal Magnolia Flower Lung–Clearing Decoction)

Long Dan Xie Gan Tang (龙胆泻肝汤 Gentian Liver–Draining Decoction) [for liver fire]

Huang Qin Hua Shi Tang (黄芩滑石汤 Scutellaria and Talcum Decoction) [for spleen–stomach damp–heat]

Wen Fei Zhi Liu Dan (温肺止流丹 Lung–Warming Nose–Drying Elixir) [for lung qi vacuity cold]

Shen Ling Bai Zhu San (参苓白朮散 Ginseng, Poria, and White Atractylodes Powder) [for spleen–stomach vacuity]

Single Medicinals:

Bai Zhi (白芷 Dahurian angelica, Angelicae Dahuricae Radix)

Cang Er Zi (苍耳子 xanthium, Xanthii Fructus)

Xin Yi (辛夷 magnolia flower, Magnoliae Flos)

Xi Xin (细辛 asarum, Asari Herba)

Stomach Pain

1. Vacuity pain of the stomach

Formulas:

Huang Qi Jian Zhong Tang (黄芪建中汤 Astragalus Center–Fortifying Decoction)

Xiao Jian Zhong Tang (小建中汤 Minor Center–Fortifying Decoction)

Single Medicinals:

Dang Shen (党参 Codonopsis, Codonopsis Radix)

Huang Qi (黄芪 Astragalus, Astragali Radix)

Bai Zhu (白术 White atractylodes, Atractylodis Macrocephalae Rhizoma)

Shan Yao (山药 Dioscorea, Dioscoreae Rhizoma)

Gan Cao (甘草 Licorice, Glycyrrhizae Radix)

Yi Tang (饴糖 Malt sugar, Maltosum)

2. Qi pain of the stomach

Formulas:

Chai Hu Shu Gan San (柴胡疏肝散 Bupleurum Liver–Coursing Powder)

Jin Ling Zi San (金铃子散 Toosendan Powder)

Chen Xiang Jiang Qi Tang (沉香降气汤 Aquilaria Qi–Downbearing Decoction)

Single Medicinals:

Chuan Lian Zi (川楝子 Toosendan, Toosendan Fructus)

Wu Yao (乌药 Lindera, Linderae Radix)

Mu Xiang (木香 Costusroot, Aucklandiae Radix)

Sha Ren (砂仁 Amomum, Amomi Fructus)

Zhi Qiao (Ke) (枳壳 Bitter orange, Aurantii Fructus)

Xiang Fu (香附 Cyperus, Cyperi Rhizoma)

Chen Pi (陈皮 Tangerine peel, Citri Reticulatae Pericarpium)

Li Zhi He (荔枝核 Litchee pit, Litchi Semen)

Tan Xiang (檀香 Sandalwood, Santali Albi Lignum)

Mei Gui Hua (玫瑰花 Rose, Rosae Rugosae Flos)

Fo Shou (佛手 Buddha's hand, Sacrodactylis Fructus)

3. Cold pain of the stomach

Formulas:

Liang Fu Wan (良附丸 Lesser Galangal and Cyperus Pill)

Fu Zi Li Zhong Wan (附子理中丸 Aconite Center–Rectifying Pill)

Single Medicinals:

Sheng Jiang (生姜 Fresh ginger, Zingiberis Rhizoma Recens)

Gan Jiang (干姜 Dried ginger, Zingiberis Rhizoma)

Gao Liang Jiang (高良姜 Lesser galangal, Alpiniae Officinarum Rhizoma)

Wu Zhu Yu (吴茱萸 Evodia, Evodiae Fructus)

Fu Zi (附子 Aconite, Aconiti Radix Lateralis Praeparata)

Rou Gui (肉桂 Cinnamon bark, Cinnamomi Cortex)

Hua Jiao (花椒 Zanthoxylum, Zanthoxyli Pericarpium)

Bai Dou Kou (白豆蔻 Cardamom, Amomi Fructus Rotundus)

Sha Ren (砂仁 Amomum, Amomi Fructus)

Tan Xiang (檀香 Sandalwood, Santali Albi Lignum)

Cao Guo (草果 Tsaoko, Tsaoko Fructus)

Ding Xiang (丁香 Clove, Caryophylli Flos)

4. Heat pain of the stomach

Formulas:

Zuo Jin Wan (左金丸 Left–Running Metal Pill)

Single Medicinals:

Shi Gao (石膏 Gypsum, Gypsum Fibrosum)

Da Huang (大黄 Rhubarb, Rhei Radix et Rhizoma)

Huang Lian (黄连 Coptis, Coptidis Rhizoma)

Zhi Zi (栀子 Gardenia, Gardeniae Fructus)

Chuan Lian Zi (川楝子 Toosendan, Toosendan Fructus)

Zhu Ru (竹茹 Bamboo shavings, Bumbusae Caulis in Taenia)

5. Stasis pain of the stomach

Formulas:

Shi Xiao San (失笑散 Sudden Smile Powder)

Dan Shen Yin (丹参饮 Salvia Beverage)

Single Medicinals:

San Leng (三棱 Sparganium, Sparganii Rhizoma)

E Zhu (莪术 Curcuma rhizome, Curcumae Rhizoma)

Pu Huang (蒲黄 Typha pollen, Typhae Pollen)

Wu Ling Zhi (五灵脂 Squirrel's droppings, Trogopteri Faeces)

Ru Xiang (乳香 Frankincense, Olibanum)

Mo Yao (没药 Myrrh, Myrrha)

Yan Hu Suo (延胡索 Corydalis, Corydalis Rhizoma)

Chuan Lian Zi (川楝子 Toosendan, Toosendan Fructus)

6. Food stagnation stomach pain

Formulas:

Bao He Wan (保和丸 Harmony–Preserving Pill)

Zhi Shi Dao Zhi Wan (枳实导滞丸 Unripe Bitter Orange Stagnation–Abducting Pill)

Xiao Cheng Qi Tang (小承气汤 Minor Qi–Infusing Decoction)

Single Medicinals:

Mai Ya (麦芽 Barley sprout, Hordei Fructus Germinatus)

Shan Zha (山楂 Crataegus, Crataegi Fructus)

Gu Ya (谷芽 Millet sprout, Setariae Fructus Germinatus)

Shen Qu (神曲 Medicated leaven, Massa Medicata Fermentata)

Ji Nei Jin (鸡内金 Gizzard lining, Galli Gigeriae Endothelium Corneum)

Qing Pi (青皮 Unripe tangerine peel, Citri Reticulatae Pericarpium Viride)

Abdominal Pain

1. Qi stagnation abdominal pain

Formulas:

Chai Hu Shu Gan San (柴胡疏肝散 Bupleurum Liver–Coursing Powder)

Jin Ling Zi San (金铃子散 Toosendan Powder)

Single Medicinals:

Fo Shou (佛手 Buddha's hand, Sacrodactylis Fructus)

Hou Po (厚朴 Officinal magnolia bark, Magnoliae Officinalis Cortex)

Zhi Shi (枳实 Unripe bitter orange, Aurantii Fructus Immaturus)

Xiang Fu (香附 Cyperus, Cyperi Rhizoma)

Mu Xiang (木香 Costusroot, Aucklandiae Radix)

Wu Yao (乌药 Lindera, Linderae Radix)

Chen Xiang (沉香 Aquilaria, Aquilariae Lignum Resinatum)

Qing Pi (青皮 Unripe tangerine peel, Citri Reticulatae Pericarpium Viride)

Chuan Lian Zi (川楝子 Toosendan, Toosendan Fructus)

Tan Xiang (檀香 Sandalwood, Santali Albi Lignum)

Sha Ren (砂仁 Amomum, Amomi Fructus)

Yi Zhi Ren (益智仁 Alpinia, Alpiniae Oxyphyllae Fructus)

Rou Dou Kou (肉豆蔻 Nutmeg, Myristicae Semen)

2. Blood stasis abdominal pain

Formulas:

Shi Xiao San (失笑散 Sudden Smile Powder)

Dan Shen Yin (丹参饮 Salvia Beverage)

Single Medicinals:

Wu Ling Zhi (五灵脂 Squirrel's droppings, Trogopteri Faeces)

Hong Hua (红花 Carthamus, Carthami Flos)

Su Mu (苏木 Sappan, Sappan Lignum)

Gui Zhi (桂枝 Cinnamon twig, Cinnamomi Ramulus)

Tao Ren (桃仁 Peach kernel, Persicae Semen)

Yi Mu Cao (益母草 Leonurus, Leonuri Herba)

San Leng (三棱 Sparganium, Sparganii Rhizoma)

E Zhu (莪术 Curcuma rhizome, Curcumae Rhizoma)

Bai Jiang Cao (败酱草 Patrinia, Patriniae Herba)

Shan Zha (山楂 Crataegus, Crataegi Fructus)

Yan Hu Suo (延胡索 Corydalis, Corydalis Rhizoma)

3. Food accumulation abdominal pain

Formulas:

Bao He Wan (保和丸 Harmony–Preserving Pill)

Zhi Shi Dao Zhi Wan (枳实导滞丸 Unripe Bitter Orange Stagnation–Abducting Pill)

Single Medicinals:

Shan Zha (山楂 Crataegus, Crataegi Fructus)

Shen Qu (神曲 Medicated leaven, Massa Medicata Fermentata)

Mai Ya (麦芽 Barley sprout, Hordei Fructus Germinatus)

4. Blood vacuity abdominal pain

Formulas:

Shao Yao Gan Cao Tang (芍药甘草汤 Peony and Licorice Decoction)

Single Medicinals:

Dang Gui (当归 Chinese angelica, Angelicae Sinensis Radix)

Bai Shao (白芍 Paeoniae Radix Alba, white peony)

Shu Di Huang (熟地黄 Cooked rehmannia, Rehmanniae Radix Praeparata)

5. Vacuity cold abdominal pain

Formulas:

Huang Qi Jian Zhong Tang (黄芪建中汤 Astragalus Center–Fortifying Decoction)

Xiao Jian Zhong Tang (小建中汤 Minor Center–Fortifying Decoction)

Single Medicinals:

Yi Tang (饴糖 Malt sugar, Maltosum)

Ai Ye (艾叶 Mugwort, Artemisiae Argyi Folium)

6. Intestinal welling–abscess abdominal pain

Formulas:

Da Huang Mu Dan Pi Tang (大黄牡丹皮汤 Rhubarb and Moutan Decoction)

Single Medicinals:

Mu Dan Pi (牡丹皮 Moutan, Moutan Cortex)

Da Huang (大黄 Rhubarb, Rhei Radix et Rhizoma)

Tao Ren (桃仁 Peach kernel, Persicae Semen)

Chi Shao Yao (赤芍药 Red peony, Paeoniae Radix Rubra)

Da Xue Teng (大血藤 Sargentodoxa, Sargentodoxae Caulis)

Bai Jiang Cao (败酱草 Patrinia, Patriniae Herba)

Vomiting

1. Vomiting from wind–cold

Formulas:

Huo Xiang Zheng Qi San (藿香正气散 Agastache Qi–Righting Powder)

Single Medicinals:

Sheng Jiang (生姜 Fresh ginger, Zingiberis Rhizoma Recens)

Zi Su Ye (紫苏叶 Perilla leaf, Perillae Folium)

Pei Lan (佩兰 Eupatorium, Eupatorii Herba)

Huo Xiang (藿香 Patchouli, Pogostemonis Herba)

Xiang Ru (香薷 Mosla, Moslae Herba)

2. Vomiting from stomach cold

Formulas:

Li Zhong Wan (理中丸 Center–Rectifying Pill)

Xiao Ban Xia Tang (小半夏汤 Minor Pinellia Decoction)

Single Medicinals:

Wu Zhu Yu (吴茱萸 Evodia, Evodiae Fructus)

Gao Liang Jiang (高良姜 Lesser galangal, Alpiniae Officinarum Rhizoma)

Bai Dou Kou (白豆蔻 Cardamom, Amomi Fructus Rotundus)

Xiao Hui Xiang (小茴香 Fennel, Foeniculi Fructus)

Ban Xia (半夏 Pinellia, Pinelliae Rhizoma)

Gan Jiang (干姜 Dried ginger, Zingiberis Rhizoma)

Sheng Jiang (生姜 Fresh ginger, Zingiberis Rhizoma Recens)

Ding Xiang (丁香 Clove, Caryophylli Flos)

Sha Ren (砂仁 Amomum, Amomi Fructus)

Tan Xiang (檀香 Sandalwood, Santali Albi Lignum)

Cao Guo (草果 Tsaoko, Tsaoko Fructus)

Hua Jiao (花椒 Zanthoxylum, Zanthoxyli Pericarpium)

Hu Jiao (胡椒 Pepper, Piperis Fructus)

Chen Xiang (沉香 Aquilaria, Aquilariae Lignum Resinatum)

3. Vomiting from stomach heat

Formulas:

Zuo Jin Wan (左金丸 Left–Running Metal Pill) [repletion]

Mai Men Dong Tang (麦门冬汤 Ophiopogon Decoction) [yin vacuity]

Single Medicinals:

Lu Gen (芦根 Phragmites, Phragmitis Rhizoma)

Zhu Ru (竹茹 Bamboo shavings, Bumbusae Caulis in Taenia)

Huang Lian (黄连 Coptis, Coptidis Rhizoma)

Pi Pa Ye (枇杷叶 Loquat leaf, Eriobotryae Folium)

Bai Mao Gen (白茅根 Imperata, Imperatae Rhizoma)

4. Vomiting from qi stagnation

Formulas:

Ban Xia Hou Po Tang (半夏厚朴汤 Pinellia and Officinal Magnolia Bark Decoction)

Zuo Jin Wan (左金丸 Left–Running Metal Pill)

Single Medicinals:

Chen Pi (陈皮 Tangerine peel, Citri Reticulatae Pericarpium)

Zi Su Ye (紫苏叶 Perilla leaf, Perillae Folium)

Sha Ren (砂仁 Amomum, Amomi Fructus)

Shi Di (柿蒂 Persimmon calyx, Kaki Calyx)

Tan Xiang (檀香 Sandalwood, Santali Albi Lignum)

Chen Xiang (沉香 Aquilaria, Aquilariae Lignum Resinatum)

Fo Shou (佛手 Buddha's hand, Sacrodactylis Fructus)

Xuan Fu Hua (旋覆花 Inula flower, Inulae Flos)

Bai Dou Kou (白豆蔻 Cardamom, Amomi Fructus Rotundus)

Cao Dou Kou (草豆蔻 Katsumada's galangal seed, Alpiniae Katsumadai Semen)

Wu Zhu Yu (吴茱萸 Evodia, Evodiae Fructus)

Mu Xiang (木香 Costusroot, Aucklandiae Radix)

5. Vomiting from food damage

Formulas:

Bao He Wan (保和丸 Harmony–Preserving Pill)

Single Medicinals:

Mai Ya (麦芽 Barley sprout, Hordei Fructus Germinatus)

Shen Qu (神曲 Medicated leaven, Massa Medicata Fermentata)

Shan Zha (山楂 Crataegus, Crataegi Fructus)

Ji Nei Jin (鸡内金 Gizzard lining, Galli Gigeriae Endothelium Corneum)

Lai Fu Zi (莱菔子 Radish seed, Raphani Semen)

6. Vomiting from phlegm turbidity

Formulas:

Xiao Ban Xia Tang (小半夏汤 Minor Pinellia Decoction)

Ling Gui Zhu Gan Tang (苓桂术甘汤 Poria, Cinnamon Twig, White Atractylodes, and Licorice Decoction)

Single Medicinals:

Chen Pi (陈皮 Tangerine peel, Citri Reticulatae Pericarpium)

Ban Xia (半夏 Pinellia, Pinelliae Rhizoma)

Sheng Jiang (生姜 Fresh ginger, Zingiberis Rhizoma Recens)

Fu Ling (茯苓 Poria, Poria)

Xuan Fu Hua (旋覆花 Inula flower, Inulae Flos)

Huang Qin (黄芩 Scutellaria, Scutellariae Radix)

Long Dan (龙胆 Gentian, Gentianae Radix)

Diarrhea

1. Qi stagnation diarrhea

Formulas:

Tong Xie Yao Fang (痛泻要方 Pain and Diarrhea Formula)

Single Medicinals:

Mu Xiang (木香 Costusroot, Aucklandiae Radix)

Bing Lang (槟榔 Areca, Arecae Semen)

2. Cold–damp diarrhea

Formulas:

Huo Xiang Zheng Qi San (藿香正气散 Agastache Qi–Righting Powder)

Wei Ling Tang (胃苓汤 Stomach–Calming Poria Five Decoction)

Single Medicinals:

Cao Guo (草果 Tsaoko, Tsaoko Fructus)

Cao Dou Kou (草豆蔻 Katsumada's galangal seed, Alpiniae Katsumadai Semen)

Sha Ren (砂仁 Amomum, Amomi Fructus)

3. Food Stagnation diarrhea

Formulas:

Bao He Wan (保和丸 Harmony–Preserving Pill)

Zhi Shi Dao Zhi Wan (枳实导滞丸 Unripe Bitter Orange Stagnation–Abducting Pill)

Single Medicinals:

Shan Zha (山楂 Crataegus, Crataegi Fructus)

Shen Qu (神曲 Medicated leaven, Massa Medicata Fermentata)

Mai Ya (麦芽 Barley sprout, Hordei Fructus Germinatus)

4. Damp–heat diarrhea

Formulas:

Ge Gen Qin Lian Tang (葛根芩连汤 Pueraria, Scutellaria, and Coptis Decoction)

Single Medicinals:

Huang Lian (黄连 Coptis, Coptidis Rhizoma)

Huang Qin (黄芩 Scutellaria, Scutellariae Radix)

5. Spleen vacuity diarrhea

Formulas:

Shen Ling Bai Zhu San (参苓白术散 Ginseng, Poria, and White Atractylodes Powder)

Bu Zhong Yi Qi Tang (补中益气汤 Center–Supplementing Qi–Boosting Decoction)

Single Medicinals:

Bai Zhu (白朮 White atractylodes, Atractylodis Macrocephalae Rhizoma)

Shan Yao (山药 Dioscorea, Dioscoreae Rhizoma)

Fu Ling (茯苓 Poria, Poria)

Bian Dou (扁豆 Lablab, Lablab Semen Album)

Gan Cao (甘草 Licorice, Glycyrrhizae Radix)

Qian Shi (芡实 Euryale, Euryales Semen)

Lian Zi (莲子 Lotus fruit/seed, Nelumbinis Semen)

Sheng Ma (升麻 Cimicifuga, Cimicifugae Rhizoma)

Ge Gen (葛根 Pueraria, Puerariae Radix) [roasted]

Ai Ye (艾叶 Mugwort, Artemisiae Argyi Folium)

Tu Si Zi (菟丝子 Cuscuta, Cuscutae Semen)

Xian He Cao (仙鹤草 Agrimony, Agrimoniae Herba)

Yi Yi Ren (薏苡仁 Coix, Coicis Semen)

6. Spleen cold diarrhea

Formulas:

Fu Zi Li Zhong Wan (附子理中丸 Aconite Center–Rectifying Pill)

Single Medicinals:

Wu Zhu Yu (吴茱萸 Evodia, Evodiae Fructus)

Fu Zi (附子 Aconite, Aconiti Radix Lateralis Praeparata) [processed]

Sha Ren (砂仁 Amomum, Amomi Fructus)

Gan Jiang (干姜 Dried ginger, Zingiberis Rhizoma)

Hua Jiao (花椒 Zanthoxylum, Zanthoxyli Pericarpium)

Bi Bo (荜茇 Long pepper, Piperis Longi Fructus)

Gao Liang Jiang (高良姜 Lesser galangal, Alpiniae Officinarum Rhizoma)

Hu Jiao (胡椒 Pepper, Piperis Fructus)

7. Kidney yang vacuity diarrhea

Formulas:

Si Shen Wan (四神丸 Four Spirits Pill)

Single Medicinals:

Yi Zhi Ren (益智仁 Alpinia, Alpiniae Oxyphyllae Fructus)

Wu Wei Zi (五味子 Schisandra, Schisandrae Fructus)

Wu Zhu Yu (吴茱萸 Evodia, Evodiae Fructus)

Bu Gu Zhi (补骨脂 Psoralea, Psoraleae Fructus)

Constipation

1. Repletion heat constipation

Formulas:

Da Cheng Qi Tang (大承气汤 Major Qi–Infusing Decoction)

Xiao Cheng Qi Tang (小承气汤 Minor Qi–Infusing Decoction)

Tiao Wei Cheng Qi Tang (调胃承气汤 Stomach–Regulating Qi–Infusing Decoction)

Single Medicinals:

Da Huang (大黄 Rhubarb, Rhei Radix et Rhizoma)

Mang Xiao (芒硝 Mirabilite, Natrii Sulfas)

Hou Po (厚朴 Officinal magnolia bark, Magnoliae Officinalis Cortex)

Zhi Shi (枳实 Unripe bitter orange, Aurantii Fructus Immaturus)

Fan Xie Ye (番泻叶 Senna, Sennae Folium)

Lu Hui (芦荟 Aloe, Aloe)

Jue Ming Zi (决明子 Fetid cassia, Cassiae Semen)

Hu Zhang (虎杖 Bushy knotweed, Polygoni Cuspidati Rhizoma)

2. Dryness–heat constipation

Formulas:

Ma Zi Ren Wan (麻子仁丸 Cannabis Seed Pill)

Single Medicinals:

Huo Ma Ren (火麻仁 Cannabis fruit, Cannabis Fructus)

Yu Li Ren (郁李仁 Bush cherry kernel, Pruni Semen)

Dong Kui Zi (冬葵子 Mallow seed, Malvae Semen)

Tao Ren (桃仁 Peach kernel, Persicae Semen)

Gua Lou (栝楼 Trichosanthes, Trichosanthis Fructus)

Xing Ren (杏仁 Apricot kernel, Armeniacae Semen)

Zi Su Zi (紫苏子 Perilla fruit, Perillae Fructus)

Jue Ming Zi (决明子 Fetid cassia, Cassiae Semen)

Rou Cong Rong (肉苁蓉 Cistanche, Cistanches Herba)

Feng Mi (蜂蜜 Honey, Mel)

Suo Yang (锁阳 Cynomorium, Cynomorii Herba)

Hu Tao Ren (胡桃仁 Walnut, Juglandis Semen)

Dang Gui (当归 Chinese angelica, Angelicae Sinensis Radix)

Tian Men Dong (天门冬 Asparagus, Asparagi Radix)

Sang Shen (桑椹 Mulberry, Mori Fructus)

He Shou Wu (何首乌 Flowery knotweed, Polygoni Multiflori Radix)

Sheng Di Huang (生地黄 Dried/fresh rehmannia, Rehmanniae Radix Exsiccata seu Recens)

Hei Zhi Ma (黑脂麻 Black sesame, Sesami Semen Nigrum)

3. Qi constipation

Formulas:

Liu Mo Yin (六磨饮 Six Milled Ingredients Beverage)

Single Medicinals:

Chen Xiang (沉香 Aquilaria, Aquilariae Lignum Resinatum)

Bing Lang (槟榔 Areca, Arecae Semen)

Zhi Qiao (Ke) (枳壳Bitter orange, Aurantii Fructus)

4. Vacuity constipation

Formulas:

Run Chang Wan (润肠丸 Intestine–Moistening Pill)

Wu Ren Wan (五仁丸 Five Kernels Pill)

Single Medicinals:

Feng Mi (蜂蜜 Honey, Mel)

Bai Zi Ren (柏子仁 Arborvitae seed, Platycladi Semen)

Hei Zhi Ma (黑脂麻 Black sesame, Sesami Semen Nigrum)

Sheng Bai Zhu (生白术 Raw ovate atractylodes, Atractylodis Ovatae Rhizoma Crudum)

5. Vacuity cold constipation

Formulas:

Ji Chuan Jian (济川煎 Ferry Brew)

Single Medicinals:

Huo Ma Ren (火麻仁 Cannabis seed, Cannabis Semen)

Rou Cong Rong (肉苁蓉 Cstanche, Cistanches Herba)

Suo Yang (锁阳 Cynomorium, Cynomorii Herba)

6. Center qi fall constipation

Formulas:

Huang Qi Tang (黄芪汤 Astragalus Decoction)

Bu Zhong Yi Qi Tang (补中益气汤 Center–Supplementing Qi–Boosting Decoction)

Single Medicinals:

Huang Qi (黄芪 Astragalus, Astragali Radix)

Ren Shen (人参 Ginseng, Ginseng Radix)

Sheng Ma (升麻 Cimicifuga, Cimicifugae Rhizoma)

Chai Hu (柴胡 Bupleurum, Bupleuri Radix)

Ge Gen (葛根 Pueraria, Puerariae Radix)

Zhi Shi (枳实 Unripe bitter orange, Aurantii Fructus Immaturus)

Zhi Qiao (Ke) (枳壳 Bitter orange, Aurantii Fructus)

Gui Zhi (桂枝 Cinnamon twig, Cinnamomi Ramulus)

Prolapse of the Rectum

Formulas:

Yi Zi Tang (乙字汤 One Zi Decoction)

Bu Zhong Yi Qi Tang (补中益气汤 Center–Supplementing Qi–Boosting Decoction)

Single Medicinals:

Chai Hu (柴胡 Bupleurum, Bupleuri Radix)

Sheng Ma (升麻 Cimicifuga, Cimicifugae Rhizoma)

Huang Qi (黄芪 Astragalus, Astragali Radix)

Zhi Shi (枳实 Unripe bitter orange, Aurantii Fructus Immaturus)

Zhi Qiao (Ke) (枳壳 Bitter orange, Aurantii Fructus)

Jie Geng (桔梗 Platycodon, Platycodonis Radix)

Ge Gen (葛根 Pueraria, Puerariae Radix)

Wu Bei Zi (五倍子 Sumac gallnut, Galla Chinensis)

Menstrual Pain

1. Qi stagnation menstrual pain

Formulas:

Chai Hu Shu Gan San (柴胡疏肝散 Bupleurum Liver–Coursing Powder)

Single Medicinals:

Chai Hu (柴胡 Bupleurum, Bupleuri Radix)

Xiang Fu (香附 Cyperus, Cyperi Rhizoma)

Wu Yao (乌药 Lindera, Linderae Radix)

Bo He (薄荷 Mint, Menthae Herba)

Chuan Lian Zi (川楝子 Toosendan, Toosendan Fructus)

Yu Jin (郁金 Curcuma, Curcumae Radix)

Li Zhi He (荔枝核 Litchee pit, Litchi Semen)

2. Blood stasis menstrual pain

Formulas:

Ge Xia Zhu Yu Tang (膈下逐瘀汤 Infradiaphragmatic Stasis–Expelling
Decoction)

Shao Fu Zhu Yu Tang (少腹逐瘀汤 Lesser Abdomen Stasis–Expelling
Decoction)

Single Medicinals:

Chuan Xiong (川芎 Chuanxiong, Chuanxiong Rhizoma)

Dan Shen (丹参 Salvia, Salviae Miltiorrhizae Radix)

Yi Mu Cao (益母草 Leonurus, Leonuri Herba)

Tao Ren (桃仁 Peach kernel, Persicae Semen)

Hong Hua (红花 Carthamus, Carthami Flos)

Dang Gui (当归 Chinese angelica, Angelicae Sinensis Radix)

Wu Ling Zhi (五灵脂 Squirrel's droppings, Trogopteri Faeces)

Pu Huang (蒲黄 Typha pollen, Typhae Pollen)

Ru Xiang (乳香 Frankincense, Olibanum)

Mo Yao (没药 Myrrh, Myrrha)

Ze Lan (泽兰 Lycopus, Lycopi Herba)

Chi Shao Yao (赤芍药 Red peony, Paeoniae Radix Rubra)

Niu Xi (牛膝 Achyranthes, Achyranthis Bidentatae Radix)

San Leng (三棱 Sparganium, Sparganii Rhizoma)

E Zhu (莪术 Curcuma rhizome, Curcumae Rhizoma)

Gui Zhi (桂枝 Cinnamon twig, Cinnamomi Ramulus)

Shan Zha (山楂 Crataegus, Crataegi Fructus)

Yan Hu Suo (延胡索 Corydalis, Corydalis Rhizoma)

Yu Jin (郁金 Curcuma, Curcumae Radix)

Jiang Huang (姜黄 Turmeric, Curcumae Longae Rhizoma)

Ji Xue Teng (鸡血藤 Spatholobus, Spatholobi Caulis)

Shui Zhi (水蛭 Leech, Hirudo)

Mu Dan Pi (牡丹皮 Moutan, Moutan Cortex)

Qian Cao (茜草 Madder, Rubiae Radix)

Hu Po (琥珀 Amber, Succinum)

Xue Jie (血竭 Dragon's blood, Daemonoropis Resina)

3. Cold congealing menstrual pain

Formulas:

Shao Fu Zhu Yu Tang (少腹逐瘀汤 Lesser Abdomen Stasis–Expelling Decoction)

Wen Jing Tang (温经汤 Channel–Warming (Menses–Warming) Decoction)

Single Medicinals:

Rou Gui (肉桂 Cinnamon bark, Cinnamomi Cortex)

Gui Zhi (桂枝 Cinnamon twig, Cinnamomi Ramulus)

Wu Zhu Yu (吴茱萸 Evodia, Evodiae Fructus)

Ai Ye (艾叶 Mugwort, Artemisiae Argyi Folium)

Pao Jiang (炮姜 Blast–fried ginger, Zingiberis Rhizoma Praeparatum)

Wu Yao (乌药 Lindera, Linderae Radix)

4. Qi vacuity menstrual pain

Formulas:

Sheng Yu Tang (圣愈汤 Sagacious Cure Decoction)

Bu Zhong Yi Qi Tang (补中益气汤 Center–Supplementing Qi–Boosting Decoction)

Single Medicinals:

Dang Shen (党参 Codonopsis, Codonopsis Radix)

Ren Shen (人参 Ginseng, Ginseng Radix)

Huang Qi (黄芪 Astragalus, Astragali Radix)

Stirring Fetus

Stirring fetus is a disease pattern characterized by movement of the fetus, pain and a sagging sensation in the abdomen, and, in severe cases, discharge of blood via the vagina. It is a sign of possible or impending miscarriage.

1. Stirring fetus due to qi vacuity

Formulas:

Tai Yuan Yin (胎元饮 Fetal Origin Beverage)

Single Medicinals:

Ren Shen (人参 Ginseng, Ginseng Radix)

Huang Qi (黄芪 Astragalus, Astragali Radix)

Bai Zhu (白术 White atractylodes, Atractylodis Macrocephalae Rhizoma)

2. Stirring fetus due to blood vacuity

Formulas:

Tai Yuan Yin (胎元饮 Fetal Origin Beverage)

Single Medicinals:

Dang Gui (当归 Chinese angelica, Angelicae Sinensis Radix)

Bai Shao Yao (白芍药 White peony, Paeoniae Radix Alba)

Shu Di Huang (熟地黄 Cooked rehmannia, Rehmanniae Radix Praeparata)

E Jiao (阿胶 Ass hide glue, Asini Corii Colla)

3. Stirring fetus due to kidney vacuity

Formulas:

Shou Tai Wan (寿胎丸 Fetal Longevity Pill)

Single Medicinals:

Sang Ji Sheng (桑寄生 Mistletoe, Taxilli Herba)

Xu Duan (续断 Dipsacus, Dipsaci Radix)

Du Zhong (杜仲 Eucommia, Eucommiae Cortex)

Tu Si Zi (菟丝子 Cuscuta, Cuscutae Semen)

4. Stirring fetus due to blood heat

Formulas:

Bao Yin Jian (保阴煎 Yin–Safeguarding Brew)

Single Medicinals:

Huang Qin (黄芩 Scutellaria, Scutellariae Radix)

5. Stirring fetus due to qi stagnation

Single Medicinals:

Sha Ren (砂仁 Amomum, Amomi Fructus)

Zi Su Geng (紫苏梗 Perilla stem, Perillae Caulis)

Vaginal Discharge

A scant white vaginal discharge often occurs in healthy women. Only discharge that is profuse, bears an unnatural color, or gives off a malign odor is pathological.

1. Vaginal discharge from damp–heat

Formulas:

Zhi Dai Fang (止带方 Discharge–Checking Formula)

Yi Huang San (益黄散 Transforming Yellow Powder)

Si Miao San (四妙散 Mysterious Four Powder)

Single Medicinals:

Huang Bai (黄柏 Phellodendron, Phellodendri Cortex)

Ku Shen (苦参 Flavescent sophora, Sophorae Flavescentis Radix)

Ze Xie (泽泻 Alisma, Alismatis Rhizoma)

Huang Lian (黄连 Coptis, Coptidis Rhizoma)

2. Vaginal discharge from spleen vacuity

Formulas:

Wan Dai Tang (完带汤 Discharge–Ceasing Decoction)

Single Medicinals:

Bai Guo (白果 Ginkgo, Ginkgo Semen)

Bai Zhu (白朮 White atractylodes, Atractylodis Macrocephalae Rhizoma)

Cang Zhu (苍朮 Atractylodes, Atractylodis Rhizoma)

Shan Yao (山药 Dioscorea, Dioscoreae Rhizoma)

Yi Yi Ren (薏苡仁 Coix, Coicis Semen)

Qian Shi (芡实 Euryale, Euryales Semen)

Lian Zi (莲子 Lotus fruit/seed, Nelumbinis Semen)

3. Vaginal discharge from cold–damp

Formulas:

Wan Dai Tang (完带汤 Discharge–Ceasing Decoction)

Er Chen Tang (二陈汤 Two Matured Ingredients Decoction)

Single Medicinals:

Bai Zhi (白芷 Dahurian angelica, Angelicae Dahuricae Radix)

Cang Zhu (苍朮 Atractylodes, Atractylodis Rhizoma)

Bai Zhu (白朮 White atractylodes, Atractylodis Macrocephalae Rhizoma)

Ai Ye (艾叶 Mugwort, Artemisiae Argyi Folium)

Hai Piao Xiao (海螵蛸 Cuttlefish bone, Sepiae Endoconcha)

4. Vaginal discharge from kidney vacuity

Formulas:

Nei Bu Wan (内补丸 Internal Supplementation Pill)

Zhi Bai Di Huang Wan (知柏地黄丸 Anemarrhena, Phellodendron, and Rehmannia Pill)

Single Medicinals:

Long Gu (龙骨 Dragon bone, Mastodi Ossis Fossilia)

Mu Li (牡蛎 Oyster shell, Ostreae Concha)

Tu Si Zi (菟丝子 Cuscuta, Cuscutae Semen)

Sha Yuan Zi (沙苑子 Complanate astragalus seed, Astragali Complanati Semen)

Jiu Zi (韭子 Chinese leek seed, Allii Tuberosi Semen)

Lian Zi (莲子 Lotus fruit/seed, Nelumbinis Semen)

Qian Shi (芡实 Euryale, Euryales Semen)

Jin Ying Zi (金樱子 Cherokee rose fruit, Rosae Laevigatae Fructus)

Sang Piao Xiao (桑螵蛸 Mantis egg–case, Mantidis Ootheca)

Hai Piao Xiao (海螵蛸 Cuttlefish bone, Sepiae Endoconcha)

Gou Ji (狗脊 Cibotium, Cibotii Rhizoma)

Lu Rong (鹿茸 Velvet deerhorn, Cervi Cornu Pantotrichum)

Chest Pain

1. Qi vacuity chest pain

Formulas:

Sheng Mai San (生脉散 Pulse–Engendering Powder)

Ren Shen Yang Rong Tang (人参养荣汤 Ginseng Construction–Nourishing Decoction)

Single Medicinals:

Ren Shen (人参 Ginseng, Ginseng Radix)

Dang Shen (党参 Codonopsis, Codonopsis Radix)

Huang Qi (黄芪 Astragalus, Astragali Radix)

Xi Yang Shen (西洋参 American ginseng, Panacis Quinquefolii Radix)

Tai Zi Shen (太子参 Pseudostellaria, Pseudostellariae Radix)

Wu Wei Zi (五味子 Schisandra, Schisandrae Fructus)

2. Qi stagnation chest pain

Single Medicinals:

Zhi Shi (枳实 Unripe bitter orange, Aurantii Fructus Immaturus)

Zhi Qiao (Ke) (枳壳 Bitter orange, Aurantii Fructus)

Chen Xiang (沉香 Aquilaria, Aquilariae Lignum Resinatum)

Tan Xiang (檀香 Sandalwood, Santali Albi Lignum)

Wu Yao (乌药 Lindera, Linderae Radix)

3. Blood stasis chest pain

Formulas:

Xue Fu Zhu Yu Tang (血府逐瘀汤 House of Blood Stasis–Expelling Decoction)

Dan Shen Yin (丹参饮 Salvia Beverage)

Single Medicinals:

Chuan Xiong (川芎 Chuanxiong, Chuanxiong Rhizoma)

Yan Hu Suo (延胡索 Corydalis, Corydalis Rhizoma)

Yu Jin (郁金 Curcuma, Curcumae Radix)

Dan Shen (丹参 Salvia, Salviae Miltiorrhizae Radix)

Jiang Huang (姜黄 Turmeric, Curcumae Longae Rhizoma)

Wu Ling Zhi (五灵脂 Squirrel's droppings, Trogopteri Faeces)

Hong Hua (红花 Carthamus, Carthami Flos)

Bai Jiang Cao (败酱草 Patrinia, Patriniae Herba)

4. Phlegm obstruction chest pain

Formulas:

Gua Lou Xie Bai Ban Xia Tang (栝楼薤白半夏汤 Trichosanthes, Chinese Chive, and Pinellia Decoction)

Single Medicinals:

Gua Lou (栝楼 Trichosanthes, Trichosanthis Fructus)

Ban Xia (半夏 Pinellia, Pinelliae Rhizoma)

Hou Po (厚朴 Officinal magnolia bark, Magnoliae Officinalis Cortex)

Chen Pi (陈皮 Tangerine peel, Citri Reticulatae Pericarpium)

Gui Zhi (桂枝 Cinnamon twig, Cinnamomi Ramulus)

Bai Jie Zi (白芥子 White mustard, Sinapis Albae Semen)

Zhi Shi (枳实 Unripe bitter orange, Aurantii Fructus Immaturus)

Xie Bai (薤白 Chinese chive, Allii Macrostemonis Bulbus)

5. Yang vacuity chest pain

Formulas:

You Gui Wan (右归丸 Right–Restoring [Life Gate] Pill)

Shen Fu Tang (参附汤 Ginseng and Aconite Decoction)

Single Medicinals:

Fu Zi (附子 Aconite, Aconiti Radix Lateralis Praeparata)

Gui Zhi (桂枝 Cinnamon twig, Cinnamomi Ramulus)

Xie Bai (薤白 Chinese chive, Allii Macrostemonis Bulbus)

Yin Yang Huo (淫羊藿 Epimedium, Epimedii Herba)

Water Swelling

1. Exterior pattern water swelling

Formulas:

Yue Bi Jia Zhu Tang (越婢加朮汤 Spleen–Effusing Decoction Plus White Atractylodes)

Fang Ji Huang Qi Tang (防己黄芪汤 Fangji and Astragalus Decoction)

Single Medicinals:

Ma Huang (麻黄 Ephedra, Ephedrae Herba)

Gui Zhi (桂枝 Cinnamon twig, Cinnamomi Ramulus)

Fu Ping (浮萍 Duckweed, Spirodelae Herba)

Xiang Ru (香薷 Mosla, Moslae Herba)

2. Skin water

Formulas:

Wu Pi San (五皮散 Five–Peel Powder)

Single Medicinals:

Sheng Jiang Pi (生姜皮 Ginger skin, Zingiberis Rhizomatis Cortex)

Da Fu Pi (大腹皮 Areca husk, Arecae Pericarpium)

Sang Bai Pi (桑白皮 Mulberry root bark, Mori Cortex)

Wu Jia Pi (五加皮 Acanthopanax, Acanthopanacis Cortex)

3. Yang vacuity water swelling

Formulas:

Jin Gui Shen Qi Wan (金匮肾气丸 Golden Coffer Kidney Qi Pill)

Zhen Wu Tang (真武汤 True Warrior Decoction)

Single Medicinals:

Fu Zi (附子 Aconite, Aconiti Radix Lateralis Praeparata)

Rou Gui (肉桂 Cinnamon bark, Cinnamomi Cortex)

Gui Zhi (桂枝 Cinnamon twig, Cinnamomi Ramulus)

4. Qi vacuity water swelling

Formulas:

Shi Pi Yin (实脾饮 Spleen–Firming Beverage)

Shen Ling Bai Zhu San (参苓白朮散 Ginseng, Poria, and White Atractylodes Powder)

Single Medicinals:

Huang Qi (黄芪 Astragalus, Astragali Radix)

Dang Shen (党参 Codonopsis, Codonopsis Radix)

Bai Zhu (白朮 White atractylodes, Atractylodis Macrocephalae Rhizoma)

Yi Yi Ren (薏苡仁 Coix, Coicis Semen)

Fu Ling (茯苓 Poria, Poria)

5. Cold–damp water swelling

Formulas:

Wu Ling San (五苓散 Poria Five Powder)

Single Medicinals:

Gui Zhi (桂枝 Cinnamon twig, Cinnamomi Ramulus)

Fu Zi (附子 Aconite, Aconiti Radix Lateralis Praeparata)

Wu Jia Pi (五加皮 Acanthopanax, Acanthopanacis Cortex)

6. Water–damp water swelling

Formulas:

Wu Pi San (五皮散 Five–Peel Powder)

Wei Ling Tang (胃苓汤 Stomach–Calming Poria Five Decoction)

Single Medicinals:

Ze Xie (泽泻 Aalisma, Alismatis Rhizoma)

Shi Wei (石韦 Pyrrosia, Pyrrosiae Folium)

Chi Xiao Dou (赤小豆 Rice bean, Phaseoli Semen)

Wu Jia Pi (五加皮 Acanthopanax, Acanthopanacis Cortex)

Sang Bai Pi (桑白皮 Mulberry root bark, Mori Cortex)

Ze Lan (泽兰 Lycopus, Lycopi Herba)

Yi Mu Cao (益母草 Leonurus, Leonuri Herba)

Ting Li Zi (葶苈子 Lepidium/descurainiae, Lepidii/Descurainiae Semen)

Sweating Patterns

1. Spontaneous sweating

Construction–defense disharmony:
Formulas:

Gui Zhi Tang (桂枝汤 Cinnamon Twig Decoction)

Single Medicinals:

Gui Zhi (桂枝 Cinnamon twig, Cinnamomi Ramulus)

Bai Shao Yao (白芍药 White peony, Paeoniae Radix Alba)

Insufficiency of lung qi:
Formulas:

Yu Ping Feng San (玉屏风散 Jade Wind–Barrier Powder)

Mu Li San (牡蛎散 Oyster Shell Powder)

Single Medicinals:

Bai Zhu (白术 White atractylodes, Atractylodis Macrocephalae Rhizoma)

Huang Qi (黄芪 Astragalus, Astragali Radix)

Wu Wei Zi (五味子 Schisandra, Schisandrae Fructus)

Internal heat:
Single Medicinals:

Zhi Mu (知母 Anemarrhena, Anemarrhenae Rhizoma)

Shi Gao (石膏 Gypsum, Gypsum Fibrosum)

2. Night sweating from insufficiency of heart blood

Formulas:

Gan Mai Da Zao Tang (甘麦大枣汤 Licorice, Wheat, and Jujube Decoction)

Suan Zao Ren Tang (酸枣仁汤 Spiny Jujube Decoction)

Single Medicinals:

Suan Zao Ren (酸枣仁 Spiny jujube, Ziziphi Spinosi Semen)

Fu Xiao Mai (浮小麦 Light wheat, Tritici Fructus Levis)

Wu Wei Zi (五味子 Schisandra, Schisandrae Fructus)

3. Night sweating from effulgent yin vacuity fire

Formulas:

Qing Hao Bie Jia Tang (青蒿鳖甲汤 Sweet Wormwood and Turtle Shell Decoction)

Mu Li San (牡蛎散 Oyster Shell Powder)

Single Medicinals:

Di Gu Pi (地骨皮 Lycium root bark, Lycii Cortex)

Shan Zhu Yu (山茱萸 Cornus, Corni Fructus)

Ma Huang Gen (麻黄根 Ephedra root, Ephedrae Radix)

Zhi Mu (知母 Anemarrhena, Anemarrhenae Rhizoma)

Wu Mei (乌梅 Mume, Mume Fructus)

4. Desertion sweating

Formulas:

Sheng Mai San (生脉散 Pulse–Engendering Powder)

Du Shen Tang (独参汤 Pure Ginseng Decoction)

Shen Fu Tang (参附汤 Ginseng and Aconite Decoction)

Single Medicinals:

Ren Shen (人参 Ginseng, Ginseng Radix)

Fu Zi (附子 Aconite, Aconiti Radix Lateralis Praeparata)

Bai Zhu (白朮 White atractylodes, Atractylodis Macrocephalae Rhizoma)

Huang Qi (黄芪 Astragalus, Astragali Radix)

Wu Wei Zi (五味子 Schisandra, Schisandrae Fructus)

Long Gu (龙骨 Dragon bone, Mastodi Ossis Fossilia) [calcined]

Mu Li (牡蛎 Oyster shell, Ostreae Concha) [calcined]

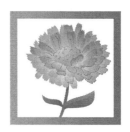

Bibliography

Pharmacopoeia of the People's Republic of China (中华人民共和国药典), Chemistry and Industry Press, Beijing. 2005.

Clinical Applications of Chinese Medical Granules (中药配方颗粒临床应用集萃), Chinese Medicine Press, Beijing. 2008.

TLC Atlas of Concentrated Granules for Prescriptions, Jiangsu Technology Press, Jiangyin, 2001.

Chinese Medicinals (*Zhong Yao Xue* 中药学), 5th ed., Shanghai Technology Press, Shanghai. 1985.

Chinese Medicinals (*Zhong Yao Xue* 中药学), 6th ed., Shanghai Technology Press, Shanghai, 1995.

Chinese Formulas (*Fang Ji Xue* 方剂学), Shanghai Technology Press, Shanghai, 2006.

Chinese Medicinals (*Zhong Yao Xue* 中药学), 7th ed., People's Medical Publishing House, Beijing, 2002.

Chinese Medicinals (*Zhong Yao Xue* 中药学), 7th ed., Hunan Technology Press, Hunan, 2004

Clinical Chinese Medicinals (*Lin Chuang Zhong Yao Xue* 临床中药学), Chinese Medicine Press, Beijing, 2004.

Chinese Medicinals (*Zhong Yao Xue* 中藥學), Zhiyin Press, Taipei, 2003.

Chinese Formulas (*Fang Ji Xue* 方劑學), Zhiyin Press, Taipei, 1996.

Chinese Medicinals (*Zhong Yao Xue* 中药学), People's Medical Publishing House, Beijing, 2000.

Chinese Medicinals (Zhong Yao Xue 中药学), 7th ed., Chinese Medicine Press, Beijing, 2002.

Chinese Medicinals (Zhong Yao Xue 中药学), People's Medical Publishing House, Beijing, 2005 (2nd ed.).

Chinese Medicinal Processing (Zhong Yao Pao Zhi Xue 中藥炮制學), Zhiyin Press, Taipei, 2002.

Great Dictionary of Chinese Medicine (Zhong Yi Da Ci Dian 中医大辞典), People's Medical Publishing House, Beijing, 2006 (2nd ed.).

Great Encyclopedia of Chinese Medicinals (Zhong Yao Da Ci Dian 中药大辞典), Shanghai Technology Press, Shanghai, 1975.

Sea of Chinese Medicinals (Zhong Hua Yao Hai 中华药海), Harbin Press, Harbin, 1994.

Conference on Chinese Medical Product Differentiation, China Medical University, Oct 8th, 2009.

Chang Hsien-Cheh, personal correspondence, 2008-2010.

Chang Hen-Hong, personal correspondence, 2006.

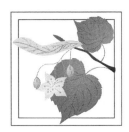

General Index

C

ACUPOINT POCKET REFERENCE
by Bob Flaws
ISBN 0-936185-93-7
ISBN 978-0-936185-93-4

ACUPUNCTURE, CHINESE MEDICINE & HEALTHY
WEIGHT LOSS   Revised Edition
by Juliette Aiyana, L. Ac.
ISBN 1-891845-61-6
ISBN 978-1-891845-61-1

ACUPUNCTURE & IVF
by Lifang Liang
ISBN 0-891845-24-1
ISBN 978-0-891845-24-6

ACUPUNCTURE FOR STROKE REHABILITATION
Three Decades of Information from China
by Hoy Ping Yee Chan, et al.
ISBN 1-891845-35-7
ISBN 978-1-891845-35-2

ACUPUNCTURE PHYSICAL MEDICINE: An
Acupuncture Touchpoint Approach to the Treatment
of Chronic Pain, Fatigue, and Stress Disorders
by Mark Seem
ISBN 1-891845-13-6
ISBN 978-1-891845-13-0

AGING & BLOOD STASIS: A New Approach to TCM
Geriatrics
by Yan De-xin
ISBN 0-936185-63-6
ISBN 978-0-936185-63-7

AN ACUPUNCTURISTS GUIDE TO MEDICAL RED
FLAGS & REFERRALS
by Dr. David Anzaldua, MD
ISBN 1-891845-54-3
ISBN 978-1-891845-54-3

BETTER BREAST HEALTH NATURALLY with
CHINESE MEDICINE
by Honora Lee Wolfe & Bob Flaws
ISBN 0-936185-90-2
ISBN 978-0-936185-90-3

BIOMEDICINE: A TEXTBOOK FOR PRACTITIONERS
OF ACUPUNCTURE AND ORIENTAL MEDICINE
by Bruce H. Robinson, MD Second Edition
ISBN 1-891845-62-4
ISBN 978-1-891845-62-8

THE BOOK OF JOOK: Chinese Medicinal Porridges
by Bob Flaws
ISBN 0-936185-60-6
ISBN 978-0-936185-60-0

CHANNEL DIVERGENCES Deeper Pathways of the
Web
by Miki Shima and Charles Chase
ISBN 1-891845-15-2
ISBN 978-1-891845-15-4

CHINESE MEDICAL OBSTETRICS
by Bob Flaws
ISBN 1-891845-30-6
ISBN 978-1-891845-30-7

CHINESE MEDICAL PALM IS TRY: Your Health in
Your Hand
by Zong Xiao-fan & Gary Liscum
ISBN 0-936185-64-3
ISBN 978-0-936185-64-4

CHINESE MEDICAL PSYCHIATRY: A Textbook and
Clinical Manual
by Bob Flaws and James Lake, MD
ISBN 1-845891-17-9
ISBN 978-1-845891-17-8

CHINESE MEDICINAL TEAS: Simple, Proven, Folk
Formulas for Common Diseases & Promoting Health
by Zong Xiao-fan & Gary Lis cum
ISBN 0-936185-76-7
ISBN 978-0-936185-76-7

CHINESE MEDICINAL WINES & ELIXIRS
by Bob Flaws Revised Edition
ISBN 0-936185-58-9
ISBN 978-0-936185-58-3

CHINESE PEDIATRIC MASSAGE THERAPY: A
Parent's & Practitioner's Guide to the Prevention &
Treatment of Childhood Illness
by Fan Ya-li
ISBN 0-936185-54-6
ISBN 978-0-936185-54-5

CHINESE SCALP ACUPUNCTURE
by Jason Jishun Hao & Linda Lingzhi Hao
ISBN 1-891845-60-8
ISBN 978-1-891845-60-4

CHINESE SELF-MASSAGE THERAPY: The Easy
Way to Health
by Fan Ya-li
ISBN 0-936185-74-0
ISBN 978-0-936185-74-3

THE CLASSIC OF DIFFICULTIES: A Translation of
the Nan Jing
translation by Bob Flaws
ISBN 1-891845-07-1
ISBN 978-1-891845-07-9

A CLINICIAN'S GUIDE TO USING GRANULE
EXTRACTS
by Eric Brand
ISBN 1-891845-51-9
ISBN 978-1-891845-51-2

A COMPENDIUM OF CHINESE MEDICAL MEN-
STRUAL DISEASES
by Bob Flaws
ISBN 1-891845-31-4
ISBN 978-1-891845-31-4

CONCISE CHINESE MATERIA MEDICA
by Eric Brand and Nigel Wiseman
ISBN 0-912111-82-8
ISBN 978-0-912111-82-7

CONTEMPORARY GYNECOLOGY: An Integrated
Chinese-Western Approach
by Lifang Liang
ISBN 1-891845-50-0
ISBN 978-1-891845-50-5

CONTROLLING DIABETES NATURALLY WITH
CHINESE MEDICINE
by Lynn Kuchinski
ISBN 0-936185-06-3
ISBN 978-0-936185-06-2

CURING ARTHRITIS NATURALLY WITH CHINESE
MEDICINE
by Douglas Frank & Bob Flaws
ISBN 0-936185-87-2
ISBN 978-0-936185-87-3

CURING DEPRESSION NATURALLY WITH
CHINESE MEDICINE
by Rosa Schnyer & Bob Flaws
ISBN 0-936185-94-5
ISBN 978-0-936185-94-1

CURING FIBROMYALGIA NATURALLY WITH
CHINESE MEDICINE
by Bob Flaws
ISBN 1-891845-09-8
ISBN 978-1-891845-09-3

CURING HAY FEVER NATURALLY WITH CHINESE
MEDICINE
by Bob Flaws
ISBN 0-936185-91-0
ISBN 978-0-936185-91-0

CURING HEADACHES NATURALLY WITH
CHINESE MEDICINE
by Bob Flaws
ISBN 0-936185-95-3
ISBN 978-0-936185-95-8

CURING IBS NATURALLY WITH CHINESE
MEDICINE
by Jane Bean Oberski
ISBN 1-891845-11-X
ISBN 978-1-891845-11-6

CURING INSOMNIA NATURALLY WITH CHINESE
MEDICINE
by Bob Flaws
ISBN 0-936185-86-4
ISBN 978-0-936185-86-6

CURING PMS NATURALLY WITH CHINESE
MEDICINE
by Bob Flaws
ISBN 0-936185-85-6
ISBN 978-0-936185-85-9

DISEASES OF THE KIDNEY & BLADDER
by Hoy Ping Yee Chan, et al.
ISBN 1-891845-37-3
ISBN 978-1-891845-35-6

THE DIVINE FARMER'S MATERIA MEDICA: A
Translation of the Shen Nong Ben Cao
translation by Yang Shouz-zhong
ISBN 0-936185-96-1
ISBN 978-0-936185-96-5

DUI YAO: THE ART OF COMBINING CHINESE
HERBAL MEDICINALS
by Philippe Sionneau
ISBN 0-936185-81-3
ISBN 978-0-936185-81-1

ENDOMETRIOSIS, INFERTILITY AND TRADITIONAL
CHINESE MEDICINE: A Layperson's Guide
by Bob Flaws
ISBN 0-936185-14-7
ISBN 978-0-936185-14-9

THE ESSENCE OF LIU FENG-WU'S GYNECOLOGY
by Liu Feng-wu, translated by Yang Shou-zhong
ISBN 0-936185-88-0
ISBN 978-0-936185-88-0

EXTRA TREATISES BASED ON INVESTIGATION &
INQUIRY: A Translation of Zhu Dan-xi's Ge Zhi Yu Lun
translation by Yang Shou-zhong
ISBN 0-936185-53-8
ISBN 978-0-936185-53-8

FIRE IN THE VALLEY: TCM Diagnosis & Treatment of
Vaginal Diseases
by Bob Flaws
ISBN 0-936185-25-2
ISBN 978-0-936185-25-5

FULFILLING THE ESSENCE:
A Handbook of Traditional & Contemporary
Treatments for Female Infertility
by Bob Flaws
ISBN 0-936185-48-1
ISBN 978-0-936185-48-4

FU QING-ZHU'S GYNECOLOGY
trans. by Yang Shou-zhong and Liu Da-wei
ISBN 0-936185-35-X
ISBN 978-0-936185-35-4

GOLDEN NEEDLE WANG LE-TING: A 20th Century
Master's Approach to Acupuncture
by Yu Hui-chan and Han Fu-ru, trans. by Shuai Xue-
zhong
ISBN 0-936185-78-3
ISBN 978-0-936185-78-1

A HANDBOOK OF CHINESE HEMATOLOGY
by Simon Becker
ISBN 1-891845-16-0
ISBN 978-1-891845-16-1

A HANDBOOK OF TCM PATTERNS & THEIR
TREATMENTS
Second Edition
by Bob Flaws & Daniel Finney
ISBN 0-936185-70-8
ISBN 978-0-936185-70-5

A HANDBOOK OF TRADITIONAL CHINESE
DERMATOLOGY
by Liang Jian-hui, trans. by Zhang Ting-liang
& Bob Flaws
ISBN 0-936185-46-5
ISBN 978-0-936185-46-0

A HANDBOOK OF TRADITIONAL CHINESE
GYNECOLOGY
by Zhejiang College of TCM, trans. by Zhang Ting-
liang & Bob Flaws
ISBN 0-936185-06-6 (4th edit.)
ISBN 978-0-936185-06-4

A HANDBOOK of TCM PEDIATRICS
by Bob Flaws
ISBN 0-936185-72-4
ISBN 978-0-936185-72-9

THE HEART & ESSENCE OF DAN-XI'S METHODS
OF TREATMENT
by Xu Dan-xi, trans. by Yang Shou-zhong
ISBN 0-926185-50-3
ISBN 978-0-936185-50-7

HERB TOXICITIES & DRUG INTERACTIONS: A
Formula Approach
by Fred Jennes with Bob Flaws
ISBN 1-891845-26-8
ISBN 978-1-891845-26-0

IMPERIAL SECRETS OF HEALTH & LONGEVITY
by Bob Flaws
ISBN 0-936185-51-1
ISBN 978-0-936185-51-4

INSIGHTS OF A SENIOR ACUPUNCTURIST
by Miriam Lee
ISBN 0-936185-33-3
ISBN 978-0-936185-33-0

INTEGRATED PHARMACOLOGY: Combining Modern
Pharmacology with Chinese Medicine
by Dr. Greg Sperber with Bob Flaws
ISBN 1-891845-41-1
ISBN 978-0-936185-41-3

INTRODUCTION TO THE USE OF PROCESSED
CHINESE MEDICINALS
by Philippe Sionneau
ISBN 0-936185-62-7
ISBN 978-0-936185-62-0

KEEPING YOUR CHILD HEALTHY WITH CHINESE
MEDICINE
by Bob Flaws
ISBN 0-936185-71-6
ISBN 978-0-936185-71-2

THE LAKESIDE MASTER'S STUDY OF THE PULSE
by Li Shi-zhen, trans. by Bob Flaws
ISBN 1-891845-01-2
ISBN 978-1-891845-01-7

MANAGING MENOPAUSE NATURALLY WITH
CHINESE MEDICINE
by Honora Lee Wolfe
ISBN 0-936185-98-8
ISBN 978-0-936185-98-9

MASTER HUA'S CLASSIC OF THE CENTRAL VISCERA
by Hua Tuo, trans. by Yang Shou-zhong
ISBN 0-936185-43-0
ISBN 978-0-936185-43-9

THE MEDICAL I CHING: Oracle of the Healer Within
by Miki Shima
ISBN 0-936185-38-4
ISBN 978-0-936185-38-5

MENOPAIUSE & CHINESE MEDICINE
by Bob Flaws
ISBN 1-891845-40-3
ISBN 978-1-891845-40-6

MOXIBUSTION: A MODERN CLINICAL HANDBOOK
by Lorraine Wilcox
ISBN 1-891845-49-7
ISBN 978-1-891845-49-9

MOXIBUSTION: THE POWER OF MUGWORT FIRE
by Lorraine Wilcox
ISBN 1-891845-46-2
ISBN 978-1-891845-46-8

A NEW AMERICAN ACUPUNCTURE By Mark Seem
ISBN 0-936185-44-9
ISBN 978-0-936185-44-6

PLAYING THE GAME: A Step-by-Step Approach
to Accepting Insurance as an Acupuncturist
by Greg Sperber & Tiffany Anderson-Hefner
ISBN 3-131416-11-7
ISBN 978-3-131416-11-7

POCKET ATLAS OF CHINESE MEDICINE
Edited by Marne and Kevin Ergil
ISBN 1-891845-59-4
ISBN 978-1-891845-59-8

POINTS FOR PROFIT: The Essential Guide to Practice
Success for Acupuncturists   5th Fully Edited Edition
by Honora Wolfe with Marilyn Allen
ISBN 1-891845-25-X
ISBN 978-1-891845-25-3

PRINCIPLES OF CHINESE MEDICAL ANDROLOGY:
An Integrated Approach to Male Reproductive and
Urological Health by Bob Damone
ISBN 1-891845-45-4
ISBN 978-1-891845-45-1

PRINCE WEN HUI's COOK: Chinese Dietary Therapy
By Bob Flaws & Honora Wolfe
ISBN 0-912111-05-4
ISBN 978-0-912111-05-6

THE PULSE CLASSIC: A Translation of the Mai Jing
by Wang Shu-he, trans. by Yang Shou-zhong
ISBN 0-936185-75-9
ISBN 978-0-936185-75-0

THE SECRET OF CHINESE PULSE DIAGNOSIS
by Bob Flaws
ISBN 0-936185-67-8
ISBN 978-0-936185-67-5

SECRET SHAOLIN FORMULAS FOR THE
TREATMENT OF EXTERNAL INJURY
by De Chan, trans. by Zhang Ting-liang & Bob Flaws
ISBN 0-936185-08-2
ISBN 978-0-936185-08-8

STATEMENTS OF FACT IN TRADITIONAL CHINESE
MEDICINE   Revised & Expanded
by Bob Flaws
ISBN 0-936185-52-X
ISBN 978-0-936185-52-1

STICKING TO THE POINT: A Step-by-Step Approach
to TCM Acupuncture Therapy   2 Condensed Books
by Bob Flaws & Honora Wolfe
ISBN 1-891845-47-0
ISBN 978-1-891845-47-5

A STUDY OF DAOIST ACUPUNCTURE
by Liu Zheng-cai
ISBN 1-891845-08-X
ISBN 978-1-891845-08-6

THE SUCCESSFUL CHINESE HERBALIST
by Bob Flaws and Honora Lee Wolfe
ISBN 1-891845-29-2
ISBN 978-1-891845-29-1

THE SYSTEMATIC CLASSIC OF ACUPUNCTURE &
MOXIBUSTION: A translation of the Jia Yi Jing
by Huang-fu Mi, trans. by Yang Shou-zhong &
Charles Chace
ISBN 0-936185-29-5
ISBN 978-0-936185-29-3

THE TAO OF HEALTHY EATING: DIETARY
WISDOM ACCORDING TO CHINESE MEDICINE
by Bob Flaws Second Edition
ISBN 0-936185-92-9
ISBN 978-0-936185-92-7

TEACH YOURSELF TO READ MODERN MEDICAL CHINESE
by Bob Flaws
ISBN 0-936185-99-6
ISBN 978-0-936185-99-6

TEST PREP WORKBOOK FOR BASIC TCM THEORY
by Zhong Bai-song
ISBN 1-891845-43-8
ISBN 978-1-891845-43-7

TEST PREP WORKBOOK FOR THE NCCAOM BIOMEDICINE MODULE: Exam Preparation & Study Guide
by Zhong Bai-song
ISBN 1-891845-34-9
ISBN 978-1-891845-34-5

TREATING PEDIATRIC BED-WETTING WITH ACUPUNCTURE & CHINESE MEDICINE
by Robert Helmer
ISBN 1-891845-33-0
ISBN 978-1-891845-33-8

TREATISE on the SPLEEN & STOMACH: A Translation and annotation of Li Dong-yuan's Pi Wei Lun
by Bob Flaws
ISBN 0-936185-41-4
ISBN 978-0-936185-41-5

THE TREATMENT OF CARDIOVASCULAR ISEASES WITH CHINESE MEDICINE
by Simon Becker, Bob Flaws & Robert Casañas, MD
ISBN 1-891845-27-6
ISBN 978-1-891845-27-7

THE TREATMENT OF DIABETES MELLITUS WITH CHINESE MEDICINE
by Bob Flaws, Lynn Kuchinski & Robert Casañas, M.D.
ISBN 1-891845-21-7
ISBN 978-1-891845-21-5

THE TREATMENT OF DISEASE IN TCM, Vol. 1: Diseases of the Head & Face, Including Mental & Emotional Disorders New Edition
by Philippe Sionneau & Lü Gang
ISBN 0-936185-69-4
ISBN 978-0-936185-69-9

THE TREATMENT OF DISEASE IN TCM, Vol. II: Diseases of the Eyes, Ears, Nose, & Throat
by Sionneau & Lü
ISBN 0-936185-73-2
ISBN 978-0-936185-73-6

THE TREATMENT OF DISEASE IN TCM, Vol. III: Diseases of the Mouth, Lips, Tongue, Teeth & Gums
by Sionneau & Lü
ISBN 0-936185-79-1
ISBN 978-0-936185-79-8

THE TREATMENT OF DISEASE IN TCM, Vol IV: Diseases of the Neck, Shoulders, Back, & Limbs
by Phi lippe Sion neau & Lü Gang
ISBN 0-936185-89-9
ISBN 978-0-936185-89-7

THE TREATMENT OF DISEASE IN TCM, Vol V: Diseases of the Chest & Abdomen
by Philippe Sionneau & Lü Gang
ISBN 1-891845-02-0
ISBN 978-1-891845-02-4

THE TREATMENT OF DISEASE IN TCM, Vol VI: Diseases of the Urogential System & Proctology
by Phi lippe Sion neau & Lü Gang
ISBN 1-891845-05-5
ISBN 978-1-891845-05-5

THE TREATMENT OF DISEASE IN TCM, Vol VII: General Symptoms
by Philippe Sion neau & Lü Gang
ISBN 1-891845-14-4
ISBN 978-1-891845-14-7

THE TREATMENT OF EXTERNAL DISEASES WITH ACUPUNCTURE & MOXIBUSTION
by Yan Cui-lan and Zhu Yun-long, trans. by Yang Shou-zhong
ISBN 0-936185-80-5
ISBN 978-0-936185-80-4

THE TREATMENT OF MODERN WESTERN MEDICAL DISEASES WITH CHINESE MEDICINE
by Bob Flaws & Philippe Sionneau
ISBN 1-891845-20-9
ISBN 978-1-891845-20-8

UNDERSTANDING THE DIFFICULT PATIENT: A Guide for Practitioners of Oriental Medicine
by Nancy Bilello, RN, L.ac.
ISBN 1-891845-32-2
ISBN 978-1-891845-32-1

WESTERN PHYSICAL EXAM SKILLS FOR PRACTITIONERS OF ASIAN MEDICINE
by Bruce H. Robinson & Honora Lee Wolfe
ISBN 1-891845-48-9
ISBN 978-1-891845-48-2

YI LIN GAI CUO (Correcting the Errors in the Forest of Medicine)
by Wang Qing-ren
ISBN 1-891845-39-X
ISBN 978-1-891845-39-0

70 ESSENTIAL CHINESE HERBAL FORMULAS
by Bob Flaws
ISBN 0-936185-59-7
ISBN 978-0-936185-59-0

160 ESSENTIAL CHINESE READY-MADE MEDICINES
by Bob Flaws
ISBN 1-891945-12-8
ISBN 978-1-891945-12-3

630 QUESTIONS & ANSWERS ABOUT CHINESE HERBAL MEDICINE: A Work book & Study Guide
by Bob Flaws
ISBN 1-891845-04-7
ISBN 978-1-891845-04-8

260 ESSENTIAL CHINESE MEDICINALS
by Bob Flaws
ISBN 1-891845-03-9
ISBN 978-1-891845-03-1

750 QUESTIONS & ANSWERS ABOUT ACUPUNCTURE Exam Preparation & Study Guide
by Fred Jennes
ISBN 1-891845-22-5
ISBN 978-1-891845-22-2